STEM CELLS 1-ON-1

7 QUESTIONS YOU SHOULD ASK WHEN CONSIDERING REGENERATIVE MEDICINE

A CONSUMER'S GUIDE

MIKE VAN THIELEN, PhD

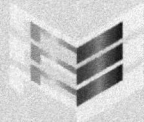

THE VERITY PRESS

Author: Dr. Mike Van Thielen
Title: Stem Cells 1-On-1
ISBN: 978-0-578-52806-9
Category: REFERENCE / Consumer Guides

Publisher: The Verity Press
Division of Devinno Technologies, LLC.

....

STEM CELLS 1-ON-1

7 QUESTIONS YOU SHOULD ASK WHEN
CONSIDERING REGENERATIVE MEDICINE

A CONSUMER'S GUIDE

MIKE VAN THIELEN, PhD

THE VERITY PRESS

TABLE OF CONTENTS

ENDORSEMENTS

"Incredible guy. If not for Dr. Mike, I wouldn't be running right now. I'd be injured on the sidelines not able to train for the Tokyo 2020 Olympics. He has become a key person in my life. He is one of those few special people that is going above and beyond what a normal doctor or business person would do. He motivates people and gives them the confidence they need to achieve their goals and dreams. I'm one of them. We have formed a special relationship that keeps growing, and I'm excited about us working together."

— Curtis Mitchell, Team USA Track & Field
2013 World Championship Bronze Medalist
2014 U.S. National Champion

"In working with many physicians and elite professional athletes over the last decade, Dr. Van Thielen is the FIRST doctor I have worked with that falls into both of those categories. His dedication to maintaining his health and body while facilitating the healing of his patients' bodies is inspiring. Dr. Mike Van Thielen has a natural and cutting-edge approach to healing and his patients see amazing success as a result of his continued innovation and dedication. Dr. Mike is also one of the most inspiring and charismatic keynote speakers I have witnessed on stage."

— Dr. Kristofer Chaffin
Doctor to professional athletes and consultant
to entrepreneurs and doctors

"I am 78 years old and received stem cell treatment for peripheral neuropathy and left knee pain. The neuropathy symptoms I was experiencing prior to my treatment were shooting and burning pains in my feet, extending up towards my knees. I had difficulty walking and was unable to walk barefoot, which was something I loved to do. I was also constantly shaking my hands because of numbness and tingling sensations. Six months after I received my stem cell treatment, my symptoms had improved over 50% already. I'm now able to walk barefoot and the tingling and numbness in my hands is almost completely gone. My knee has also improved. I only have occasional pain in my knee from the arthritis versus the high intensity pain I was experiencing prior to treatment."

– Margaret Melotz
Patient

"I am a nurse practitioner who works for Neo Matrix Medical. At the time of this writing, I received MSC's in both my knees roughly a week ago. In high school, I played as a midfielder for my hometown of Caracas, Venezuela. I have worked as a paramedic and as a nurse in busy emergency rooms in California, New Jersey and Florida for 17 years. Subsequently, my knees have taken a toll with multiple injuries as well as wear and tear over the years. After my allograft injections and SoftWave treatment last week, my knees feel like I turned back time about 20 years! Both knees feel great and I can't wait to see the final results. I cannot wait to get back to my old exercise habits."

– Luis Gomez
Patient, Licensed Nurse Practitioner

"I came to know Dr. Mike while researching stem cell therapy to possibly address Alzheimer's disease. I was leading a Health Ministry at our church and preparing presentations on Alzheimer's and Stem Cells at the time. I went to a seminar by Dr. Mike who did an excellent job of describing stem cell therapy as well as the procedures his company, Neo Matrix Medical, utilizes to maximize the health benefits. I then scheduled myself for stem cell therapy for August 29, 2018, to address my severe Sciatica. I had rejected surgery. It has now been 8 months and the results have been absolutely amazing. In addition to a full recovery from my sciatica, three other sources of pain have also vanished. Dr. Mike is a remarkable person and has built a fabulous regenerative medicine clinic. I have referred several people so far and all those who went are happy with their pain reduction and increased body function."

– Richard C. Moessner
President, Process Measurement
Systems Consulting, Inc. (Ret.)
Editorial Board, Elsevier Press,
Process Control and Quality, (Ret.)
Leader, Christian Health Ministry, Palm Coast Florida

"Dr. Mike is one of the most committed and brightest people I know. He accomplishes anything he puts his mind to and has an eye for great opportunities. In just a few short years, he has launched Neo Matrix Medical from a start-up to one of the most respected names in regenerative medicine. Dr. Mike is an outstanding communicator and public speaker. He naturally inspires and motivates any audience."

– Chip Van Vurst
CEO of BioStem Terchnologies, Inc.
Race Car Driver
Philanthropist

"I'm a 68-year-old maintenance worker suffering from neuropathy and COPD. I have had neuropathy with symptoms including burning, tingling, and pain from my toes to right above my knees. I was in terrible pain all the time. I felt as though there were burning blisters on my legs. I couldn't even touch my shin bones. My COPD caused me to cough constantly during conversation, have shortness of breath and the need to clear my throat all the time.

I had been to numerous doctors that all said there was nothing more they could do besides continue to take pain medication. I saw an article from Neo Matrix Medical and decided to come in for a consultation and give the treatment a try.

Two and a half months after my treatment I am mostly pain free in my legs and feet. The burning and blistering feeling has gone away and I can even use a washcloth on my legs. I'm able to do things I haven't done for a long time. My COPD has gotten much much better as well. I'm m now able to have a conversation without constantly coughing and clearing my throat.

My quality of life is so much better after my treatment at Neo Matrix Medical."

– Ron Abel
Patient

"In a time where health care is complicated and people are left wondering what choices they have Dr. Mike brings solutions to a broken system! Dr. Mike is changing the industry of healthcare with breakthrough science to let patients function to the best of their ability."

– Dr. Alexander Greaux
Owner - Aventura Wellness & Rehabilitation Center
Former Therapist MIAMI HEAT (NBA)

"I'm an emergency room doctor in Daytona Beach. I came to Neo Matrix Medical because I have had a bilateral ligament tear in my elbow for 25 years due to my competitive swimming career in college. Ever since this injury it has been impossible for me to swim the breaststroke. The surgery to correct this injury is called the Tommy John surgery but this surgery at my age has a mixed track record.

So, I did my research on stem cell therapy. I knew I did not want PRP because it's not very effective. The research on the mesynchymal stem cells indicated this approach would be far superior to PRP. The product and procedures at Neo Matrix Medical seemed the best choice for me.

Since my injury was chronic, the most I was hoping for was pain reduction in my everyday activities and working out. But much to my surprise, a little more than three months later, there was a complete resolution of the tear as seen on the MSK ultrasound done in the office. My function is back to where I was 25 years ago, and no pain at all!

After seeing my results, I referred my son for a torn ligament in his ankle and my dad for his both knees. I then referred my wife who suffered with chronic low back pain, and RA (Rheumatoid Arthritis). She has done very well. This treatment gave her back her life. She is able to sit for long periods of time without discomfort now and do some activities she did at college as well. I'm a believer in the regenerative medicine therapies offered at Neo Matrix Medical."

– Terry Livingston, MD
Emergency room physician

"As a retired Major-General, I enjoy playing tennis, swimming and working out. My right shoulder was giving me more and more trouble and I decided to visit the doctor. He said it was arthritis and gave me a cortisone injection but that didn't help at all. An MRI showed rotator cuff tears and the orthopedic doctor recommended a reversed shoulder replacement surgery but indicated I probably wouldn't play tennis again. Therefore, I looked for another option and ended up receiving allograft injections in my shoulder at Neo Matrix Medical. 4 months after the treatment I was totally pain-free and playing tennis again. It's been two years now and my shoulder still feels great. Dr. Mike and his team are simply excellent and care for their patients."

– Story Stevens
Retired Major-General
Veteran WWII, Korea and Vietnam

"I received stem cell-based treatment at Neo Matrix Medical for neuropathy. I was diagnosed with neuropathy about 8 years ago. I was experiencing throbbing pain, numbness and swelling in my feet. I also had balance problems. I was told I just had to live with it.

Eight months after my treatment, I had no more pain or swelling in my feet. The numbness disappeared and I now can feel the massage therapist touching my legs and feet. My balance also has improved drastically as I now can move straight down the hallway and I no longer need to hold on to the rails when I use the stairs.

I experienced additional benefits from the treatment also, including improved memory and strength. I'm able to pick up my grandchildren, play and move my harp again and use the foot pedals while playing the organ in church. My condition has improved 100%".

– Judy Brown
Patient

"I am 30 years old and have been dealing with a lot of hip pain since 2014, with the pain level at 9-10/10. I have limitations when getting out of a chair, I have to walk with a cane, and I am in pain all the time. I have seen over 20 different doctors, and orthopedists. I have also had two failed surgeries.

I was treated at Neo Matrix Medical for my both hips and my low back. Today I am walking without my cane. My pain level is down to a 4-5/10. My range of motion is normal again, and I'm able to get back to the things I love to do, including glass blowing and teaching. My condition continues to improve and I hope all my pain will resolve soon."

– Mark Crnkovich
Patient

"I got to know Mike as an inspiring motivational speaker in the Regenerative Medicine arena, working to help countless people to get treatments for devastating conditions like neuropathy, and preventing knee and hip replacements by endorsing stem cell-based treatments to shift peoples' mind from sick-care to healthcare. At the same time, Mike took the 'make it or break it' task to break several swimming records. He trained hard and DID it. What a great accomplishment and demonstration of dedication and strength. Dr. Mike, you are an inspiration for all of us."

– Felix Amon
Serial Entrepreneur in the Regenerative Medical Space

"Dr. Mike is fantastic! He is a nice and humble man and his Team at Neo Matrix Medical took excellent care of me. I received allograft injections and SoftWave therapy for my lower back and left knee. The treatment went smooth and was very professional. I feel so much better. I recommend anyone to contact Dr. Mike and seek help. He's a pro in regenerative medicine and swimming too. He knows how to make you strong again and help you achieve anything you'll want in life."

– Pinklon Thomas
2-Time World Heavyweight Boxing
Champion and author of 'Back From the Edge of Hell'

"In my efforts to assist a major client in the Middle East to provide advanced medical care to its citizens, I focused on Regenerative Medicine and in particular Stem Cell-based Therapies, as it showed promise in the treatment of a variety of endemic ills that plague this client's country, its citizens and the region. I was fortunate enough to make contact with Dr. Mike Van Thielen and his clinic. Not only a technical leader in science, he also has an uncommon ability to connect with patients, carefully explaining the procedure and expected results, giving the patient confidence. As a naturalized US citizen, he has adopted and now exudes the American Dream—innovation and results. His story is fascinating and inspiring."

– John Middleton
Retired US Army officer / 30 years in the Middle East
President - Pathfinder Security, LLC

"I have known Dr. Mike for over 8 years now. He has always been a loyal friend and a true professional in all aspects of his life. He puts 110% into everything he sets out to do or accomplish. From Swimming competitions all over the world, in which he excels, to his leadership at Neo Matrix Medical. I trusted him as a patient with physical therapy, acupuncture and trigger point injections, and with stem cell-based therapy at Neo Matrix Medical. The allograft injections prevented me to have surgery for a torn rotator cuff. A biceps dislodgement that was not repairable with conventional surgery also healed. I now have approximately 95% of the original usage of this arm because of the stem cell procedure. It has been a pleasure knowing him over these last years, both professionally and socially."

– Sharon B Phelps
Neighbor, friend, patient and client

"Dr. Mike is an amazing person of high character. His enthusiasm made me feel excited about my procedure. As a world-class athlete himself, he understands the pain that athletes go through. He has the knowledge of figuring out what's going on and how to make things better"

– Ron Dixon
NY Giants, Super Bowl XXXV
NFL Record Holder & Co-Host of iHeartradio's
Meriweather Dixon Show

"Dr. Mike is a cool cat. He's a legit pro athlete who belongs with us in the WSA World Sports Alumni. He is a topnotch physician who's been helping my friends recover from injuries. I'm looking forward to my medicinal signaling cell therapy and SoftWave treatments at his facility."

– **Brandon Meriweather**
Host of the IHeartRadio's Meriweather Dixon show.
NFL Pro Bowler for Patriots, Redskins and Giants
and All American for the Miami Hurricanes

"Finally. A Stem Cells 101 book that will turn anyone that is clueless into an expert overnight. Dr. Mike Van Thielen proves why he is a leading authority on Regenerative Medicine. Read this book once and it will completely alter your paradigm on modern medicine."

– **Charlie Williams**
CEO World Sports Alumni

"Mike Van Thielen, Ph.D. is a leading force in bringing advanced stem cell-based therapies to the market. He is a proven trailblazer and thought leader on improving technology and the best approaches to helping patients maximize the benefits of regenerative medicine applications. It's been insightful working with Dr. Mike on developing custom protocols to individualize supplement programs to enhance patient and athlete outcomes. Working side by side with him has allowed me to see that he is a visionary, patient advocate, accomplished author, great speaker, successful businessman and world-class athlete...a true renaissance man of our times!"

– **George Collins**
Owner - Life Extension Nutrition Center, Orlando

INTRODUCTION

We live in a miraculous age. The technology of the first 19 years of the 21st-century approaches that of the technology seen in the original Star Trek series or even the movie 'Back to the Future'.

Medicine and health care are no different. The reality of our today is that humanity has enjoyed more advancements in healthcare in the first 19 years of the 21st century than the entire 20th century.

As technology continues to advance, it becomes more and more practical to merge damaged human tissue with synthetic devices like computer chips in our bodies in an effort to forestall the debilitating and deleterious effects of aging. Sound like science fiction? Science fiction is much closer to science fact than you think.

For over 15 years, medicine has been able to install computer chips in the brains of Parkinson's patients in order to correct their debilitating disease. Children with deafness can get cochlear implant's installed into their brains, allowing them to hear. Bionic limbs today have the potential to operate with greater efficiency, strength and ability than biological limbs, just like Steve Austin in the $6 million man.

However, if the idea of becoming a modern-day cyborg is not your cup of tea, have no fear. Medicine has something for you too. MSCs (formerly known as Mesenchymal Stem Cells and currently and correctly referred to as Medicinal Signaling Cells) are at the center of attention in the field of Regenerative Medicine. These MSCs along with essential bio-active molecules, such as growth factors, cytokines, collagens, Hyaluronic acid, miRNA (micro-RNA), exosomes, and scaffolding have shown the potential to repair, renew and re-engineer almost any tissue or cell in the human body.

When these MSCs were first introduced to the public, there was a moral and ethical dilemma with their sourcing. But that is not the case today since the most potent MSCs are now sourced from birth tissues such as placenta and umbilical cord tissue.

Today, the most innovative allografts have shown beneficial in the treatment of conditions such as arthritis, soft tissue injuries, neuropathies, eye conditions, chronic wounds, diabetic ulcers, E.D. (erectile dysfunction) and some autoimmune conditions. Scientists agree that these MSCs and allografts are the future of medicine.

People today, especially our elderly, suffer and are in pain. Their function is impaired, they have a limited range of motion and strength, they have balance and walking issues, lack endurance, and feel fatigued.

People's pain and medical condition not only cost them thousands of dollars over the years to manage but more importantly, they miss out on many opportunities.

When we ask people: "If you wish you could do just one thing without your pain or medical condition, what would it be?" the answers include: walking without pain, walking without a cane or walker, walking the dog around the block, playing golf and tennis, fishing, dancing swimming and working out, enjoying the outdoors, traveling, and playing with the grandkids. A lot of grandparents can get on the floor with the grandkids but are unlikely to get up again.

Our most precious commodities are time and health. It's time to regain control of your health.

Our Current Health Care System

Many experts, and also patients, believe that our current healthcare system is broken.

Here are some statistics from the World Health Organization (WHO):

1. Americans spend more than 17% of each dollar on healthcare.

   For example, if we look at big companies like Ford or G.M., they spend more money on the healthcare of their employees each day than on the parts they need to manufacture cars.

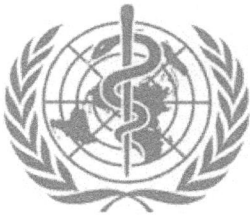

2. The U.S. ranks #37 in the world for overall health.

   This is unacceptable. We do rank number 1 for crisis care. That means acute care or emergency room care. So, if you break a leg or you are in a car accident and end up in the Emergency Room, you are in the best country in the world. However, crisis care accounts for less than 10% of overall healthcare. That means we are not helping the other 90% of people or patients. We are not taking care of people with chronic pain, arthritis, inflammatory diseases, autoimmune conditions, neurological conditions and neuropathies, etc.

3. Americans make up 5-6% of the global population, yet that small percentage consumes 50-75% of all the pharmaceutical drugs produced on this planet. We swallow more than 80% of all the painkillers, with 259 million prescriptions per year.

Let's simply face the facts and agree that our health care system in the U.S. in broken. So maybe you should consider Regenerative Medicine.

Regenerative Medicine

Regenerative medicine is an emerging branch of medicine with the goal of restoring organ and/or tissue function for patients with serious injuries or chronic diseases in which the body's own response is not effective to restore functional tissue. A growing crisis in organ transplantation and an aging population have driven a search for new and alternative therapies. There are approximately 90,000 patients on the U.S. transplant waiting list. In addition, there are a wide array of major unmet medical needs that might be addressed by regenerative technologies.

New and current Regenerative Medicine applications can use 'stem cells' to create living and functional tissues to regenerate and repair tissue and organs in the body that are damaged due to age, disease and congenital defects. Stem cells have the power to go to these damaged areas and regenerate new cells and tissues by performing a repair and a renewal process, restoring functionality. Regenerative medicine has the potential to provide a solution to failing or impaired tissues.

While some believe the therapeutic potential of 'stem cells' has been overstated, an analysis of the potential benefits of stem cells based therapies indicates that 128 million people in the United States alone may benefit with the largest impact on patients with Cardiovascular disorders

(5.5 million), autoimmune disorders (35 million) and diabetes (16 million U.S. patients and more than 217 million worldwide). U.S. patients with other disorders likely to benefit include osteoporosis (10 million), severe burns (0.3 million), spinal cord injuries (0.25 million).

Source: M.E. Furph, "Principles of Regenerative Medicine" (2008)

The "Father" of Stem Cells

Arnold I. Caplan is a Ph.D. Physiological Chemistry and Post-doctoral fellow from The Johns Hopkins University Medical School. He currently is a Professor, Department of Biology AND Director, Skeletal Research Center at Case Western Reserve University, Cleveland, Ohio.

He received many Honors & Awards, including the Lifetime Achievement Award, National Center for Regenerative Medicine, August 2015. He also published over 400 related scientific articles.

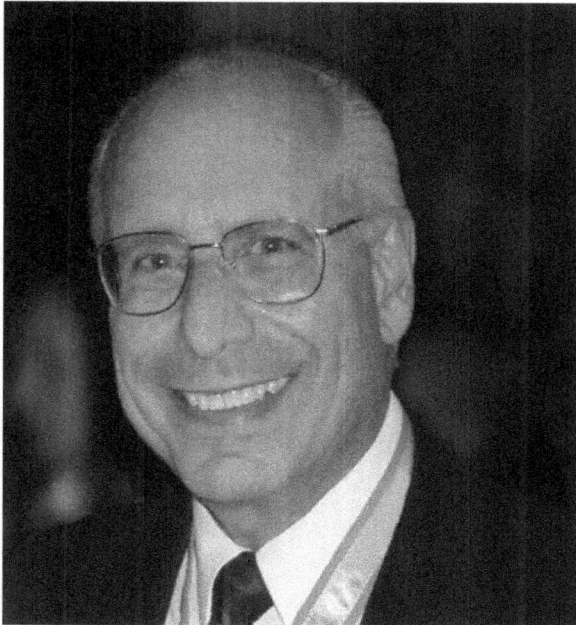

Stem Cells – A Misnomer?

Let's discuss the mechanism of action of these stem cells.

The Initial School of Thought, regarding the mechanism of action of these MSCs, was that they could replicate and differentiate into any specialized cell in our body and therefore replace and renew different tissues and cells in the body.

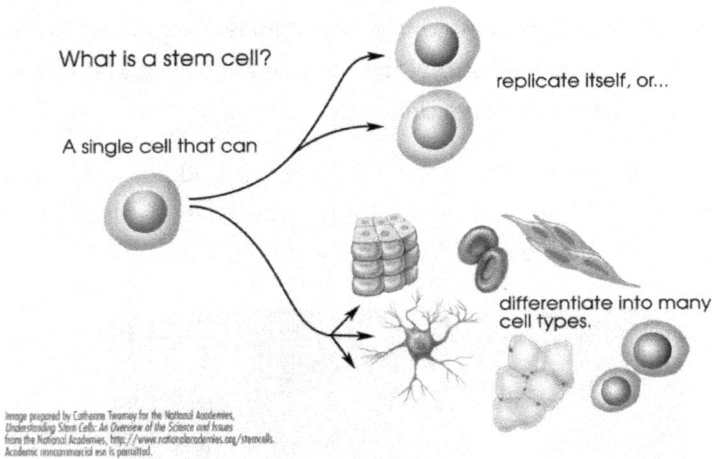

What is a stem cell?

A single cell that can

replicate itself, or...

differentiate into many cell types.

Image prepared by Catherine Twomey for the National Academies, Understanding Stem Cells: An Overview of the Science and Issues from the National Academies, http://www.nationalacademies.org/stemcells. Academic noncommercial use is permitted.

Therefore, Arnold I. Caplan named these cells Mesenchymal Stem Cells (MSCs).

Recent research into the mechanism of action of these MSCs now shows that these MSCs may not necessarily be differentiating, but rather work by stimulating the body to heal and regenerate itself through paracrine signaling, a fact that caused the father of the MSCs, Arnold Caplan, PhD, to rename MSCs to Medicinal Signaling Cells.

Robert Hariri, MD, PhD Co-founder and president, Human Longevity Cellular Therapeutics, and founder, chief scientific officer, Celgene cellular therapeutics stated in reference to MSCs: "These cells are not simply replacement parts-they are master orchestrators of processes in the organs and tissues that restart functional renovation and regeneration of those tissues."

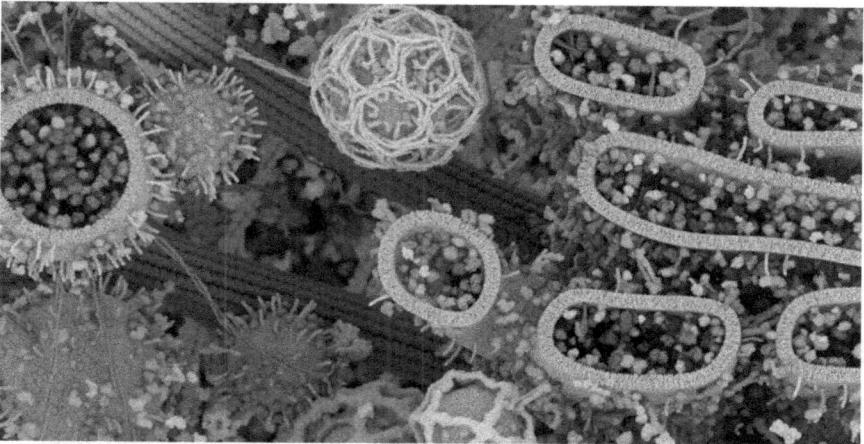

Their magic lies not in their ability to become and replace different tissues and cells, but in their production of trophic factors, bioactive molecules produced in response to the environment in which the cells find themselves. These chemicals aid in the repairing of tissue and the recruitment of new blood vessels to support oxygen and nutrient flow to the area and decrease inflammation. So, it's not the cells themselves that work their magic. It's the bio-active molecules that the cells secrete that have the medicinal properties for the body to heal and repair itself.

This new perspective on the mechanism of action of these MSC's effects the correct terminology to be used.

We should try to avoid terms such as Mesenchymal Stem Cells, Stem Cells, and live cells because they may be inaccurate and misleading when talking about Tissue Engineering. We will use the correct terminology, including Regenerative Medicine, MSCs as in Medicinal Signaling Cells, and Allograft or Allograft injections. Allografts are simply human tissues, or more specifically: "an allograft is a tissue graft from a donor of the same species as the recipient but not genetically identical."

MSCs are found throughout the entire body. They live in a specific area of each tissue, a place called the stem cell niche, where they remain dormant for long periods of time until disease or injury activates them to initiate tissue repair.

MSCs exist in many tissues as dormant cells, known as a Pericytes (peri means "around" and cyte means "cell"). Pericytes hold tight to capillaries, the smallest blood vessels that exist throughout the entire body. When the body signals an injury or inflammation, pericytes are recruited to help repair and heal tissues, at which point they become activated MSCs.

Caplan states: "MSC's are multifactorial site-specific sensors with genetically wired molecular responses. The management of innate regenerative potential is what they do."

In a fetus, inflammation in response to injury is minimized while regeneration is maximized. Scar tissue is not formed. In an adult, inflammation in response to injury is heightened, regeneration is stunted, and scar formation is emphasized. MSCs increase the regeneration phase of healing while decreasing inflammation and scar formation.

CHAPTER 1

SCIENTIFIC RESEARCH ON MSC'S

C ontrary to common belief, these MSCs have been studied for decades and thousands and thousands of scientific research articles have been published in peer-reviewed medical journals all over the world. Scientists agree that these MSCs are the future of medicine.

In the graph below, you can see the number of publications per year for the different types of stem cells. Just note that since 2015, the type of stem cells with the most publications are MSCs.

Year-Over-Year Comparison of Stem Cell Scientific Publications, by Stem Cell Type

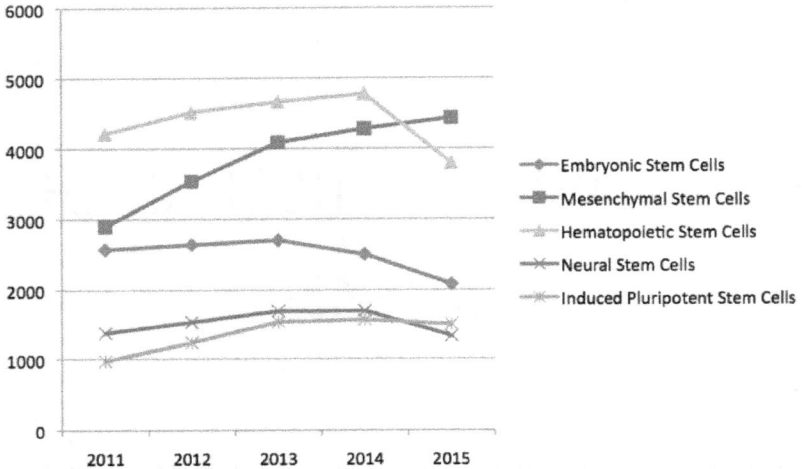

If we look at the statistics below and look at the graph on the upper left, we see that the number of scientific publications has significantly increased every year. Actually, 2/3's of all the research has been done in the last 7-8 years and that's since 1976 when these MSCs were first discovered by Friedenstein et al.

If we look closely, we can note that since 2015, more than 4000 scientific research articles were published on MSCs alone. That's far more research than any other topic in science or medicine.

The graph on the top right shows the increase in the number of clinical trials each year, and the pie chart shows the medical conditions that are being researched.

Mesenchymal Stem Stell Research: Statistics

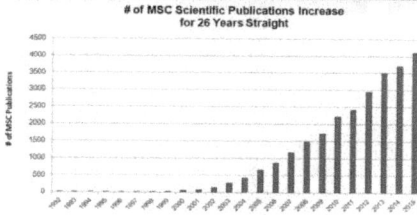

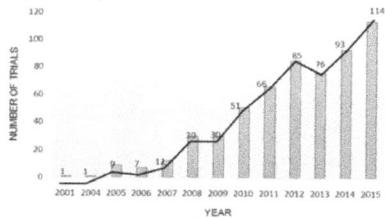

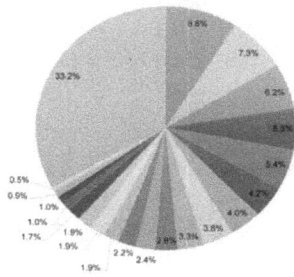

Current Research Areas of MSCs Include:

Developmental Human Biology (previously constrained by practical, moral & ethical dilemma), especially the fields of cancer and the study of birth defects.

Transplantation as we seek means to create unlimited supplies of tissues and organs that restore function without immune-suppression and tissue matching.

Gene Therapy: Genetic signaling aimed at prompting desired and necessary biochemical processes to achieve long term expression and therapeutic effect.

The 'immortal' proliferative capacity of MSCs could overcome the problems of loss and insufficient expression of a gene, cell, tissue, organ, system and your whole organism, which gene therapy procedures currently face.

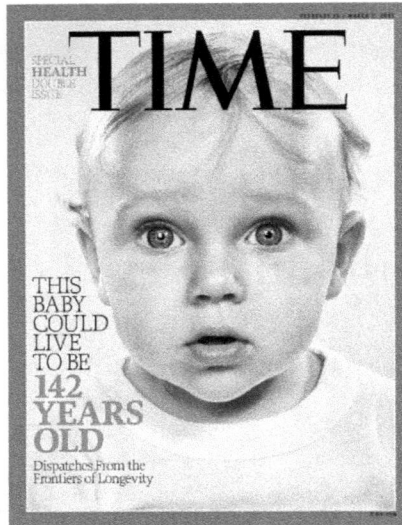

Did you know that Google now processes over 3.5 billion searches per day and 1.2 trillion searches per year? That is a massive amount of searches, especially when put into the context of there being approximately 7.4 billion people on earth.

Cell Therapy is searched 750K times a month, which is a massive number. However, the world has not really woken up to stem cell therapy yet. When it does, the monthly search volume will skyrocket to 10 or 20 times the number of searches there are today. We are truly on the ground floor as providers and clients of regenerative medicine therapies.

Instead of just managing your symptoms with drugs, injections and surgeries, you should consider options in regenerative medicine applications that are available today. Without any of the harmful adverse reactions of conventional medicine approaches, regenerative medicine puts the body in the right conditions AND provides the body with the right tools (allografts containing bio-active molecules) for the body to repair, heal and renew itself on a cellular level. These therapies not only repair, but also renew which means they will last much longer.

CHAPTER 2

7 KEY QUESTIONS

At Neo Matrix Medical, we are a few steps ahead of the competition. Below are the 7 Key Questions you should ask before you decide on Regenerative Medicine procedures, including allograft injections. You will be glad you did.

1. Are All Essential Components For Tissue Engineering (TE) In The Product?

2. What Are The Manufacturing Standards? Is The Product Safe?

3. What Type Of Imaging Is Used To Deliver The Product Accurately To The Damaged Areas?

4. What Other Modalities Are Utilized To Ensure Optimal Results?

5. How Experienced Is The Team In Performing These Procedures?

6. Do They Operate Within The Policies Recommended By The FSMB (Federation Of State Medical Boards)?

7. How Are The Results Quantified With Their Patients?

QUESTION 1: ARE ALL ESSENTIAL COMPONENTS FOR TISSUE ENGINEERING (TE) IN THE PRODUCT?

In order to effectively repair and renew tissue, we need viable MSC's but these MSC's need the support of other essential components in the body to get the job done. These components include but are not limited to: growth factors, bio-active molecules, exosomes and scaffolding.

Growth factors (usually a protein or hormone) are important for regulating a variety of cellular processes. Growth factors typically act as signaling molecules between cells. By signaling, these growth factors are believed to activate the MSCs.

Bio-active molecules such as cytokines, HA (hyaluronic acid), exosomes, collagen types I, III, IV, V, VI and VII etc. are essential for tissue repair and engineering and carry out their own specialized functions. They are like the framer, painter, plumber, carpenter, roofer etc. in the construction or reconstruction of a home or building.

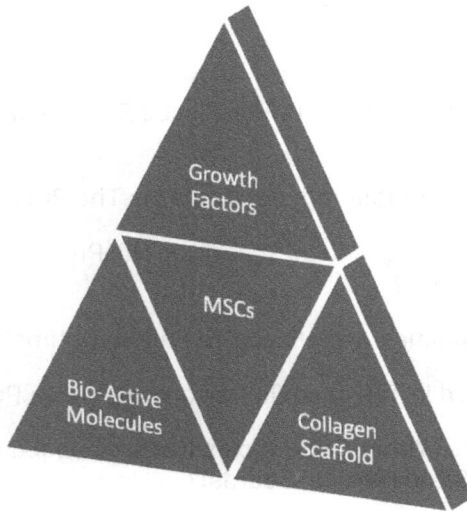

Scaffolding is the structure or framework from which the MSCs and bio-active molecules build, rebuild, repair, and re-engineer. Scaffolding is found in the ECM (extra-cellular membrane) of amniotic tissue.

More about EXOSOMES:

Exosomes are a hot topic in the field of Regenerative Medicine today. But what are exosomes and how do they contribute to tissue repair and engineering?

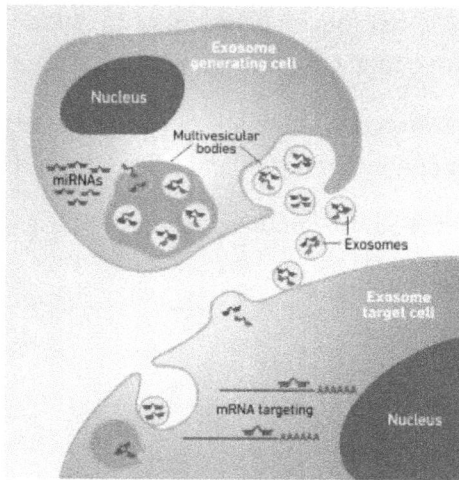

Exosomes are small vesicles that deliver bio-active molecules to the target cell.

Exosomes carry:

- Lipids
- Proteins
- GF's
- miRNA (micro)
- mRNA (messenger)

The micro RNA's are like a text or tweet (signal) and the Messenger RNA is the entire architectural blueprint that affects the DNA.

Each exosome contains a different variety of these potent miRNA. There have been 233 different miRNA identified in amniotic fluid.

Several of these exosomes promote angiogenesis. Angiogenesis is the process whereby new blood vessels are grown from the existing vascular network. Without reestablishment of the blood supply after an injury, healing will not occur. Capillary density decreases as we get older.

Based on the environment they are put in, these exosomes release the necessary components for tissue and cell repair and regeneration.

So, let's look at the various sources of these MSCs and products on the market today:

PRODUCT SOURCING

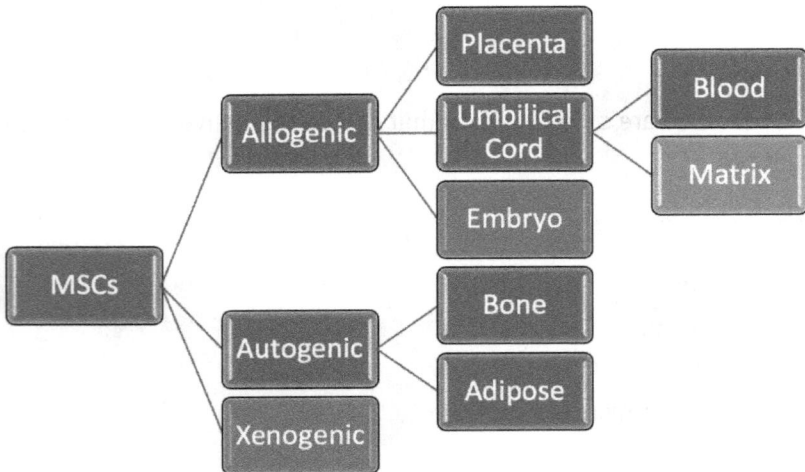

1. HUMAN EMBRYONIC TISSUE / MSCs

The use of embryonic MSCs is ILLEGAL. In addition to the moral and ethical issues that exist when harvesting MSCs from aborted fetal tissue, embryonic stem cells have been shown to cause teratomas (benign tumors) when tested on mice in laboratory settings. Embryonic MSCs are only used in research today and will NEVER be used in the therapeutic applications for humans.

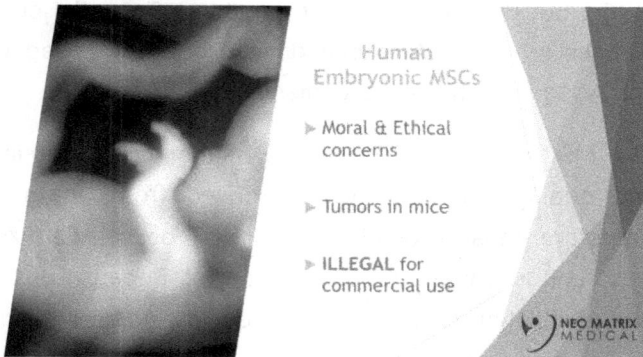

Human
Embryonic MSCs

► Moral & Ethical concerns

► Tumors in mice

► ILLEGAL for commercial use

NEO MATRIX
MEDICAL

"Embryonic MSCs once differentiated into new tissue cells, are antigenic, which means that the immune system recognizes the tissue as foreign and mounts an attack against it. Immune suppressive drugs must be administered alongside treatment with embryonic MSCs and can lead to complications.

2. AUTOGRAFTS: using your OWN tissue / MSCs

MSCs derived from bone marrow or adipose tissue of the patient are considered outdated and have many disadvantages compared to the use of MSCs from birth tissue. Here are the top 5 disadvantages:

1. The patient will have to undergo an unnecessary surgical

procedure to harvest the MSCs. Surgery not only increases risk, cost, and liability but also causes pain and often a long recovery time.

2. The other essential components for proper tissue are missing and therefore, the results may be disappointing. When we harvest MSCs from one area of the body and then relocate them to the injured or damaged area of the body, all we do is relocating the MSCs, but we are not adding anything. Essential components such as growth factors, cytokines, exosomes, collagen types III and IV, scaffolding, etc. are missing.

3. The MSCs harvested from one patient will differ in quantity and quality from the MSCs derived from another patient. Therefore, these procedures can NOT be standardized. There is no uniformity and no quality control. Because of the lack of standardization, uniformity and quality control, the FDA has issued a notice to all those practicing adipose tissue-derived stem cell-based therapies in November of 2017 stating that they have to discontinue these practices within 36 months.

4. Scientists agree that the quantity or amount of MSCs in our body drastically declines with age (refer to the graph below). When trying to harvest MSCs from the aging body, often not enough MScs are obtained. Therefore, the practitioner has to culture (amplify/multiply) these MSCs in a laboratory setting prior to administration. These cultured cells are far less effective than native cells.

5. The quality of MSCs in our aging body drastically declines with age also. Scientists explain this with the fact that the telomeres

(telomeres are the end caps of our chromosomes that protect our DNA in every cell) shorten as we age. As the telomeres shorten, the quality or the cell's ability to heal, repair, renew and regenerate drastically declines.

RESEARCH clearly demonstrates the benefits of MSCs from birth tissue (amnion, umbilical cord) versus MSCs from Bone Marrow or Adipose Tissue:

The number of stem cells in our body significantly declines with age:

Fitness of Cells with Age

As we age, our body's ability to regenerate damaged tissue decreases. This is because of the fitness of the stem cells in our bodies begin to significantly diminish over time.

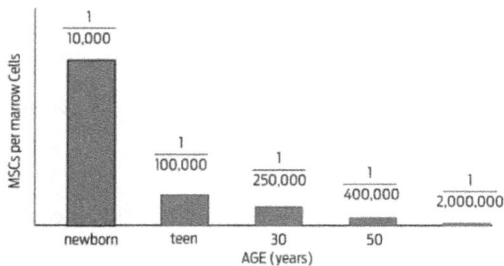

Caplan, Al. 2007. Adult Mesenchymal Stem Cells for Tissue Engineering Versus Regenerative Medicine; Journal of Cellular Physiology

"Young" MSCs obtained from birth tissue):

- Are obtained from non-invasive procedures unlike liposuction or bone marrow collection, which increase risk, cost and liability.

- Have a far greater 'fitness' level and therefore are able to replicate at greater and faster rates.

- Have a much greater and faster healing response.

- Have a higher proliferative capacity.

- Have a stronger inflammatory protective effect and a strong migratory ability toward the site of inflammation.

- Have a larger amount of different growth factors, especially bFGF 20.

- Have the ability to differentiate into adipogenic, osteogenic, chondrogenic, neural cells and Schwann cells; and help organize tendon collagen fibers and induce hepatocyte differentiation.

- Have been shown to differentiate into nervous system cells, liver, pancreas, heart, and other organs of the body.

- Are more robust. The range and level of specific cytokines are greater than those expressed by adult MSC.

- Sustain less damage from reactive oxygen species (ROS).

- Retain telomere at the highest possible length which protects them from premature loss of viability.

- Continue to express molecules with immune-modulating activity after they are extracted from the umbilical cord and able to pass this ability to their progeny. This enables the infused donor cells, whether differentiated or not, to engraft into the diseased target organ and positively modify its microenvironment to promote re-population. The infusion of immunomodulatory MSC provides a significant advantage by better overcoming host responses, providing the needed functional bridging action, and modifying the underlying pathological conditions at the basis of disease.

• Provoke little to no immune response when transplanted; cell rejection is not an issue and human leukocyte antigen (HLA) matching is not necessary (as with adult stem cells).

• Have Immunomodulatory properties: they do not pose a risk for metastasis of tumor cells and in fact, promote proteins that halt the cell cycle of cancer cells and promote tumor-suppressing genes.

All the above research facts (references listed below) are easily illustrated in the following real-life example:

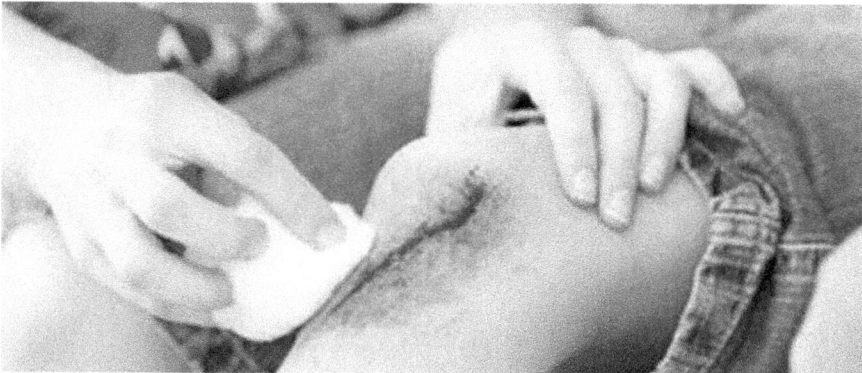

When a young child falls and cuts him/herself, how long does that cut or wound take to heal? 24-48 hours, right? What if you fall and cut yourself? Indeed, several weeks or even longer. That's because the healing properties of the young child are at its peak. The young MSCs have a far greater and faster ability to heal, repair and regenerate than our aged body MSCs.

Besides trying to harvest MSCs from the patient's own body (NOT recommended), MSCs can be obtained from birth tissue: the placenta, umbilical cord blood or umbilical cord matrix (Wharton's Jelly).

3. PLACENTAL TISSUE

Placental tissue products may contain most of the essential components for tissue engineering, including the ECM (Extra Cellular membrane) that provides scaffolding and collagens AND amniotic fluid that contains the exosomes, but lacks MSCs.

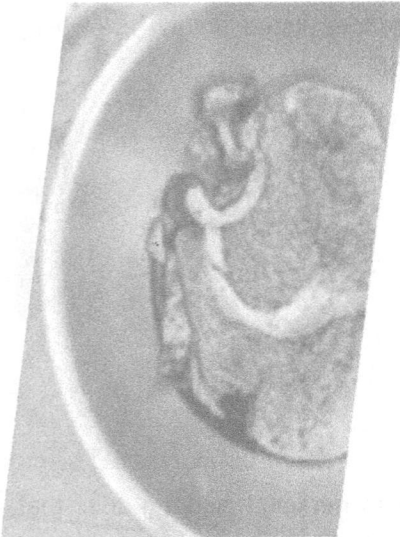

Placental Tissue
- Amnionic Membrane /ECM
  - Scaffolding
  - Collagens
- Amnionic Fluid
  - miRNA / Exosomes
- Lacks MSCs

NEO MATRIX
MEDICAL

4. UMBILICAL CORD BLOOD

Umbilical Cord Blood

- Hematopoietic cells - help form blood cells
- Chance of reaction
- NO MSCs, NO scaffolding, limited GF and cytokines, NO exosomes
- NOT fit for soft tissue modulation

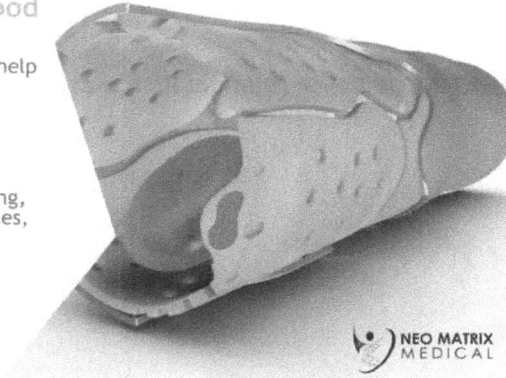

NEO MATRIX MEDICAL

Umbilical cord blood contains hematopoietic stem cells but lacks any significant number of MSCs. These products contain blood and blood fractions (increased risk of communicable disease, rejection, and allergies) and are fit to treat blood disorders and pediatric cancer but are not a good choice for soft tissue modulation.

5. UMBILICAL CORD MATRIX (WHARTON's JELLY)

Umbilical Cord Matrix (Wharton's Jelly)

CONTAINS:
- Best source of biologically young MSCs
- Lacks Scaffolding and NO exosomes

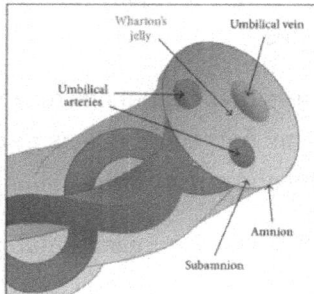

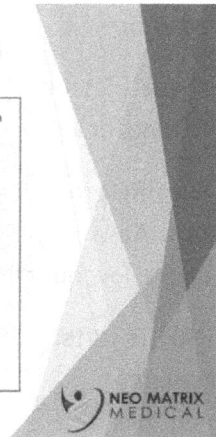

Wharton's jelly, Umbilical vein, Umbilical arteries, Amnion, Subamnion

NEO MATRIX MEDICAL

Umbilical cord matrix (Wharton's Jelly) is the best source of young MSC's but lacks scaffolding and exosomes.

6. WHAT ABOUT PRP (Platelet Rich Plasma)?

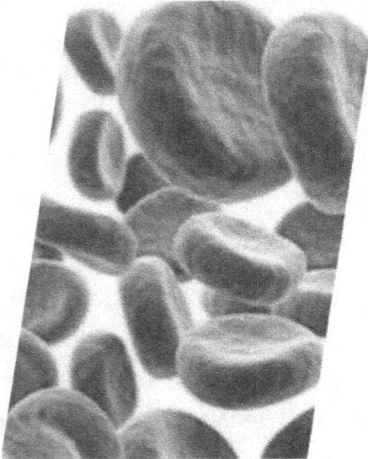

PRP
(Platelet Rich Plasma)

▶ Blood drawn from patient

▶ Platelets contain GF's, but NO MSCs, NO scaffolding, NO exosomes

▶ ONLY beneficial for younger patients and young athletes

▶ OR supplemental to Allograft

NEO MATRIX MEDICAL

The PRP procedure involves a blood draw from the patient. The vial of blood is then put in a centrifuge to separate the white and red blood cells from the platelets. The platelets are rich in GFs and injected into the injured area.

These platelets (or PRP) contains GFs, but do not contain MSCs, scaffolding, or exosomes.

The PRP procedure is ONLY beneficial for younger patients and young athletes. As we age, this procedure is less effective because we would rely on the low quantity and quality if the patient's own MSCs.

PRP is often used as a supplemental therapy to the allograft applications.

Comparison Table:

What we notice in the comparison table (below) is that each of these tissue sources or allograft products contains certain components for tissue engineering but misses other essential components.

Tissue Source	Pharma	Peripheral Blood		Placenta			Umbilical Cord		Bone Marrow	Adipose
Products	Steroid, NSAID, Synthetic HA.	Platelet Rich Plasma	Platelet Rich Plasma - Heated	Amniotic Fluid	Amniotic Matrix	Amniotic Membrane	Umbilical Cord Blood	Umbilical Cord Matrix	Bone Marrow Aspirate	Lipoaspirate
Autologous (from you)		✓							✓	✓
Allogenic (from others)				✓	✓	✓	✓	✓		
General Cytokines	✓	✓✓✓	✓✓✓	✓✓	✓✓	✓	✓	✓✓✓	✓✓	✓
Growth Factor Cytokines										
Scaffolding Cytokines					✓✓✓	✓✓✓				
Homeostatic Cytokines		✓✓✓	✓✓✓	✓✓			✓	✓✓✓	✓✓✓	✓✓✓
Mesenchymal Stem Cells (MSC)								✓✓✓	✓	✓
Viable MSCs Counts								✓✓✓		✓✓
Biologically Young Source							✓	✓✓✓		

For example:

- The umbilical cord matrix has a high amount of young MSCs but is limited in ECM material and scaffolding.

- PRP (Peripheral blood or Platelet Rich Plasma) contains no MSCs and has no scaffolding.

- Placental tissue (amnion) lacks MSCs and only has few cytokines but contains much of the ECM material and scaffolding. The amniotic fluid contains the exosomes.

- Autografts from patient's own bone marrow or adipose tissue contain MSCs but they are low in quantity and quality. These tissues are also missing the scaffolding.

At Neo Matrix Medical, we use RHEO™ from BioStem Technologies, the ONLY allograft on the market today that contains ALL ESSENTIAL COMPONENTS for Tissue Engineering.

RHEO™ contains:

- Amniotic (placental) membrane and matrix

    • ECM: scaffolding and collagens

    • Cytokines and GFs

- Amniotic fluid

    • Exosomes

    • Cytokines

- Wharton's Jelly (umbilical cord matrix)

    • Young MSCs

    • Cytokines and GF's

- HA (Hyaluronic Acid)

Conclusion:

Remember that MScs do NOT repair and heal damaged tissue, but rather the synergistic workings between all the essential components or bio-active molecules released in the environment that allow the body to repair, renew and re-engineer tissues and cells.

Other providers:

• Use an ALLOGRAFT or TISSUE PRODUCT that lacks certain essential components for effective Tissue Engineering (TE)

• Compete / Market the number of live MSCs = IRRELEVANT

- Even cells in apoptosis (cells that are dying) can release bio-active molecules in the recipient.

Neo Matrix Medical:

- RHEO™

- Contains all essential components for TE:

- Amniotic Membrane (ECM: scaffolding and collagens)

- Amniotic fluid and Exosomes

- WJ (umbilical cord matrix): Young MSCs, cytokines, GFs

- HA

QUESTION 2: WHAT ARE THE MANUFACTURING STANDARDS? IS THE PRODUCT SAFE?

About the Manufacturer

BioStem Technologies is a Publicly Traded Company (BSEM) with an FDA APPROVED LAB in South Florida. The Laboratory is a Certified ISO 5 Lab, which means that these HCT/Ps (Human Cellular Tissues and Products) are manufactured under the most rigorous and Highest Standards. This lab is Superior to all other HCT/P labs.

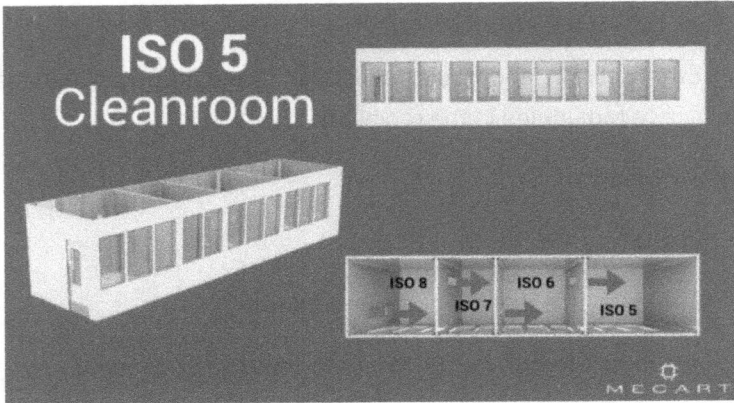

Clean Room Classification and Air Changes Per Hour

Air cleanliness is achieved by passing the air through HEPA filters. The more often the air passes through the HEPA filters, the fewer particles are left in the room air. The volume of air filtered in one hour, divided by the volume of the room gives the number of air changes per hour.

ISO Class	Average number of air changes per hour
ISO 5	240–360 air changes per hour (unidirectional airflow)
ISO 6	90–180 air changes per hour
ISO 7	30–60 air changes per hour
ISO 8	10–25 air changes per hour

Conventional building   2–4 air changes per hour

In theory, for a classified room (not just below a LAFW hood) to reach ISO5 air cleanliness, you need to enter the cleanroom via an ISO 8 (anteroom), then go through an ISO 7, followed by an ISO 6 to finally get the ISO 5.

You also can reach an ISO 5 cleanroom with 2 or 3 airlocks. The optimal layout depends on the process taking place inside the cleanroom, the size of the room, the number of people working inside, the equipment inside, etc. In addition, an ISO 5 cleanroom needs to use unidirectional airflow.

Unidirectional airflow cleanrooms use much more air than nob-directional airflow cleanrooms. High-efficiency filters are installed across the entire ceiling. The air sweeps down the room in a unidirectional way, at a velocity generally between 0.3 m/s and 0.5 m/s (meters/second), and exits through the floor, removing the airborne contamination from the room. Cleanrooms using unidirectional airflow are more expensive than non-unidirectional ones, but can comply with more stringent classifications, such as ISO 5 or lower.

At BioStem Technologies, the HCT/Ps are manufactured and tested for pathogens under these highest standards, even though not required by the FDA.

BioStem Technologies' product line is also approved for VA doctors to use at VA clinics and offices to treat our veterans.

The products contain only 3% DMSO (preservative) versus 10% in most other HCT/Ps (Human Cellular Tissues and Products). This reduces the risk for an allergic reaction to DMSO.

BioStem Technologies has four FDA 361 products on the amniotic tissue platform market, including one flowable allograft and three dehydrated membrane allografts:

- RHEO™ Flowable Allograft
- Vendaje™ Dehydrated Amnion Membrane
- Vendaje AC™ Dehydrated Amnion Membrane with Chorion and Wharton's Jelly

• Vendaje Optic™ Dehydrated Amnion Membrane for ocular repair

The products are considered extremely safe, and no adverse reactions have been reported. There is no possible rejection and no possible adverse reactions to the allografts. No blood typing is necessary for treatment.

THE PRODUCT is IN FULL COMPLIANCE WITH CURRENT FDA GUIDELINES UNDER SECTION 361 HCT/P (Human Cellular Tissues / Products):

Manufacturers and practitioners alike may be non-compliant with the current FDA regulations and recommendations. They may use a product that is not manufactured at an FDA-approved laboratory or a laboratory that is not proven to be compliant with all current FDA regulations. The practitioner may also treat patients with medical conditions that do not constitute "homologous use" and/or uses the product off-label (for the treatment of conditions not yet shown to be safe and efficacious such as cancer etc.) or for unproven stem cell-based interventions (stem cell-based therapy that lacks compelling evidence based upon scientific studies to validate treatment efficacy).

These HCT/P's (Human Cells, Tissues, and Cellular or Tissue-Based Products) are not considered drugs and therefore are not FDA-approved (except for one umbilical cord blood product that obtained approval for pediatric cancer). These products can be registered and can show compliance with the regulations set forth by the Food and Drug Administration (FDA) under 21 CFR Part 1271, section 361

Compliance:

The products we use are minimally manipulated human tissue

allografts, regulated by the Food and Drug Administration (FDA) under 21 CFR Part 1271, section 361 as HCT/Ps (Human Cells, Tissues, and Cellular or Tissue-Based Products).

At Neo Matrix Medical, we use these products for the repair, reconstruction, replacement, or supplementation of a recipient's cells or tissues that perform the same basic function or functions in the recipient as in the donor. Recipient cells or tissues may not be identical to the donor's cells or tissues but must perform one or more of the same basic functions in the recipient as the cells and tissues performed in the donor.

Compliance is important. I'm sure as a patient, you do not want to end up at a clinic that is consciously or unconsciously cutting corners, correct? Furthermore, compliance with FDA regulations improves the safety of the product and therefore mitigates the most possible risks associated with the product and procedure.

Neo Matrix Medical has addressed the FDA NOTICE re. November 2020. For a detailed insight, please refer to ADDENDUM 1.

Neo Matrix Medical also commented on the FDA warning about stem cell therapies. Please refer to ADDENDUM 2.

CONCLUSION:

The manufacturer of our Products or HCTPs (Human cellular Tissues and Products), BioStem Technologies, utilizes an FDA approved, certified ISO 5 laboratory. The manufacturing and testing standards EXCEED the FDA requirements for HCT/Ps.

The allografts are considered SAFE and NO adverse reactions have been reported.

The manufacturer is in compliance with all regulations set forth by the FDA under 21 CFR Part 1271, section 361

QUESTION 3: WHAT TYPE OF IMAGING IS USED TO DELIVER THE PRODUCT ACCURATELY TO THE DAMAGED AREAS?

Unlike many practitioners who perform 'blind' injections and don't use an imaging modality to accurately identify the damaged areas and place the product accordingly, at Neo Matrix Medical we use a 100% safe imaging modality to optimize our results.

As part of your examination before your musculoskeletal or joint injection, a diagnostic musculoskeletal (MSK) ultrasound is performed to determine the current state of the injured area and to identify the specific location of the injury. The ultrasound exam provides real-time imaging that can evaluate the health/injury of tendons, muscles, ligaments, bone, cartilage, and bursa.

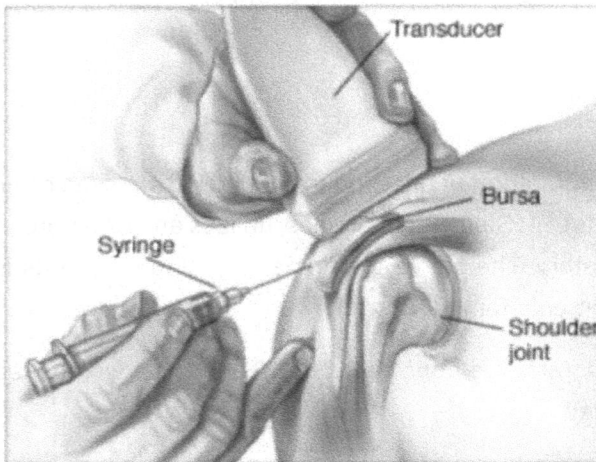

The exam consists of an ultrasound specialist using a water-based gel, as a coupling agent, and an ultrasound probe for imaging the internal structures. The sonographer will place the probe over the injured area to assess for any damage to the musculoskeletal tissue. A specific protocol will be followed for your area of concern.

Based on the amount of damage and the locations of the injuries, a detailed plan of action will be designed specifically to fit your needs.

After sterilizing the treatment area and using a local anesthetic to provide comfort, the MSK ultrasound is used for the delivery of the product to the specific site/sites of trauma.

The use of high-quality musculoskeletal ultrasonography is considered a key part of the process, particularly considering that this modality plays a central role for clinicians to effectively hit the desired targets. Optimal placement correlates with earlier and improved outcomes, making it an essential component of our regenerative therapy applications at Neo Matrix Medical.

Conclusion

The use of safe MSK Ultrasound allows for a visual diagnosis of the damaged areas and the accurate placement of the flowable allograft product in the injured areas.

QUESTION 4: WHAT OTHER MODALITIES ARE UTILIZED TO ENSURE OPTIMAL RESULTS?

Find out if the provider uses any other modalities or treatments to augment the allograft injection response. In other words, is there a synergistic treatment to obtain optimal results?

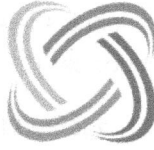

SYNERGY
BETTER TOGETHER

At Neo Matrix Medical, we have a way to ACTIVATE your OWN stem cells without surgery...

SOFTWAVE THERAPY

WHAT IS SOFTWAVE?

TRT/MTS SoftWave is a non-invasive therapeutic device using a patented breakthrough method of shock wave generation that brings unprecedented advantages to sports med and regenerative medicine in rapidly relieving chronic pain and greatly accelerating recoveries with sustaining results. This is not incremental; it is transformative and unique.

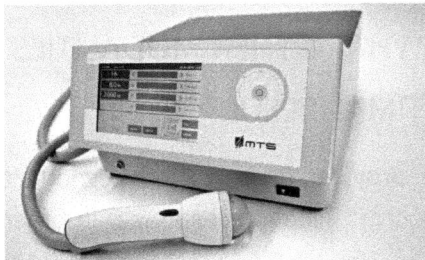

TRT/MTS OrthoGold 100 SoftWave is the only unfocused ESWT technology available, and it is scientifically validated to accomplish the following:

1. Immediately shuts down the inflammatory response at the treatment site. This has been linked to modulation of various signaling molecules, including TLR3 and NO. Results are typically immediate and sustained relief of chronic pain and release of adhesions. Restored range of motion is a common effect.

2. Sustained improvement of blood flow. This has been linked to the release of VEGF and other key growth factors and cytokines, as well as a boost in ATP, leading to neo angio/vasculogenesis at the treatment site and regenerative effect. TRT SoftWave (called MTS SparkWave in Europe) is scientifically validated to recruit and activate endogenous stem cells.

Additionally, SoftWave elicits biofeedback by which "origins of pain" can be precisely identified, serving an invaluable role in treatment effectiveness.

One to three non-invasive, atraumatic applications are all that is typically needed in many instances. SoftWave does not create, nor does it rely on, microtraumas to work. Instead, it causes cells to shed microvesicles. These micro-vesicles communicate with cells in the local environment, thereby initiating the healing cascade.

SoftWave is Unique, **Patented** and Profound. The patented unfocused electrohydraulic design of the TRT/MTS SoftWave Extracorporeal Shock Wave Therapy device brings unique and profound advantages for healing and recoveries of the human body:

•   100% atraumatic to tissue and cells

- Near-immediate pain relief in certain conditions.

- Sustained blood flow improvement.

- A wave delivery zone thousands of times larger than focused or planar designs.

- Demonstrably more efficient and effective.

- Typically, 3 applications or fewer needed.

- Real-time biofeedback provides precision guidance of application to problem origin areas. No need for imaging or trigger point references.

- Transformational vs. incremental.

- The only Unfocused Electrohydraulic ESWT available in North America, and it has FDA 510(k) clearance.

Additionally, TRT/MTS SoftWave ESWT is...

Utilized by professional sports teams AND by top medical institutions.

Top choice of many sports legends, active and retired.

Has helped thousands heal and recover in record time.

ALL SHOCK WAVE THERAPIES ARE NOT CREATED EQUAL

It's best to refer to the device as "softwave therapy" as there is much confusion regarding "shock wave therapy" since many manufacturers produce devices that do not actually create a "shock wave" yet are marketed as such. This has created confusion in the market place as well as turned off many to the technology since the mislabeled devises produce inferior results.

Knowing the different types:

It's important to understand where SoftWave fits into the big picture of the very broad term and market of "shock wave therapy."

There are 2 main categories of shock wave therapy:

1. Extracorporeal Shock Wave Therapy (ESWT), and

2. Radial Pulse Therapy (radial/ballistic devices go by many names rSWT, rESWT, RPT, EPAT, and many others). They do not produce a true "shock wave" as defined by physics (they produce a sound wave), they work on a different principle, and they are comparatively very limited as to what they can treat. Radial Pulse devices have been incorrectly referred to as "shock wave" for so long that it has stuck, though it is technically not correct.

Under the ESWT umbrella, there are 5 main categories:

1. Focused (relying on microtrauma to tissue, very small treatment zone, requires many applications over weeks/months time, and lacks the level of science that unfocused has.) Within Focused ESWT, there are three ways to produce the wave:

2. Electrohydraulic (of the 3 methods, it is demonstrated to be the most efficient and effective – see below),

3. Piezoelectric (focused and focused/planar. very little published science, typically many applications needed),

4. Electromagnetic (Scientifically shown not to be high enough energy to produce an actual shock wave, little published science, many applications needed).

5. **Unfocused (SoftWave).** TRT owns the patents to unfocused ESWT (as well as several key processes – see attachment) in North America and utilizes the electrohydraulic method to generate the waves. SoftWave (called Spark Wave & Ortho Wave in EU) is non-traumatic to tissue or cells. The treatment zone is thousands of times larger than focused or planar. it has far more published science than any other ESWT device. It also is scientifically validated to elicit a strong anti-inflammatory effect and to recruit/activate endogenous stem cells, to vascularize tissue, to promote healing, and to kill pathogens.

DEVICES THAT MARKET UNDER SHOCK WAVE THAT ARE NOT

BALLISTIC SHOCKWAVE...Do not produce a shockwave:

"Although the ballistic source investigated marketed both the terms "shock wave" and "focused' the device technically does NOT generate a focused shock wave. Electrohydraulic (EH) sources employ focusing by means of a reflector and generate chock waves at the spark source; for all settings the EH results in a shock wave at the focus. Electromagnetic and piezoelectric sources also use focusing but do NOT generate shock waves at the source.

RADIAL SHOCK WAVE THERAPY: Does not produce a shockwave at current pressure output

"It was shown that shock formation did not occur for any machine settings and that a true shock formation could be reached if the maximum initial pressure output of the device is doubled."

SOFTWAVE HAS THE SCIENCE

Patented TRT/MTS SoftWave therapy ESWT technology stands alone in the industry with quality and quantity of peer-reviewed published scientific literature validating mechanisms of action at molecular and cellular levels. All "shock wave" devices are not created equally, and one must be sure to read the scientific research applying to each specific device if one is to gain an accurate understanding of the particular device one is seeking to learn about. Many "shock wave" distributors list studies on their websites that did not use the specific device they offer but are presented as if they did. AcousTek only lists scientific studies that used TRT/MTS devices.

Review some supporting research below.

(https://neomatrixmedical.com/softwave/#research)

THE BEST KEPT SECRET IN PROFESSIONAL SPORTS

The best-kept secret in professional sports is becoming understood as the silver bullet in a team's armamentarium. Top Sports Med clinicians across the country have been quietly using SoftWave for years on injured star athletes, seeing an unprecedented acceleration of recovery times. As success after success mounts, SoftWave is now becoming more widely understood to be the profound advantage that makes a tangible difference to who plays on the field and who stays in rehab.

Some Notable Testimonials:

https://www.softwavetherapy.com/testimonials.html

Conclusion

At Neo Matrix Medical, we use our unique and innovative NEO SYNERGY protocol. We augment our allograft injections with the use of SoftWave Therapy.

This approach immediately shuts down the inflammatory response at the treatment site, which results in near-immediate pain relief in certain conditions.

Neo Synergy causes a sustained improvement of blood flow and stimulates the proliferation and differentiation of the allograft MSCs and the patient's own MSCs. This allows for effective tissue repair and healing.

We are successful in visually identifying the damaged areas with the MSK ultrasound, and locate the origin of musculoskeletal pain and referred pain with the SoftWave device. The accurate assessment and identification of the origin of pain and damaged areas allow for the correct product placement and treatment areas.

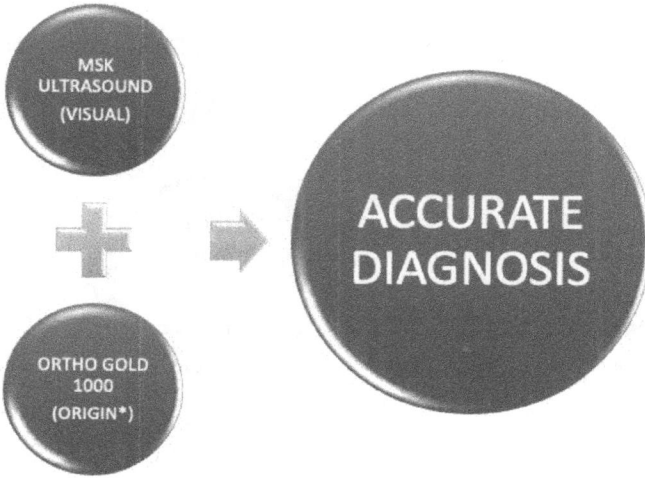

The combination of the allograft injections and SoftWave Therapy improves outcomes significantly.

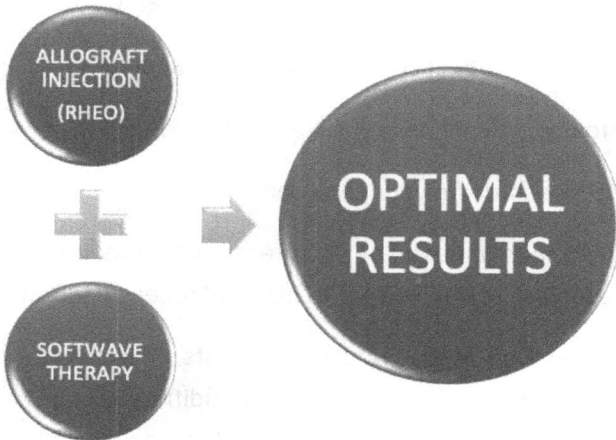

NEO SYNERGY is the name of the Treatment Protocol at Neo Matrix Medical:

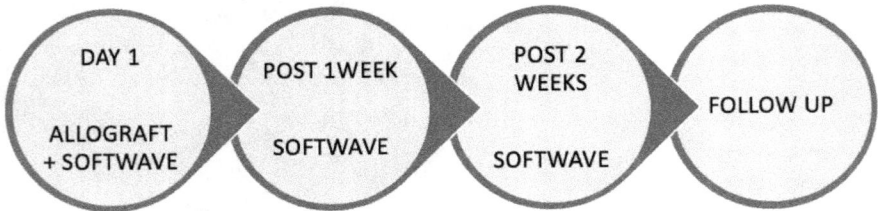

QUESTION 5: HOW EXPERIENCED IS THE TEAM IN PERFORMING THESE PROCEDURES?

When considering these Regenerative Medicine therapies, ask the provider:

- How long have you been providing these therapies?

- Do you offer other services? What's your specialty?

- How many patients have you treated?

- How successful are your outcomes?

Many physicians or health care professionals offer regenerative and 'stem cell therapies', as they call it, but have not received targeted training.

Our Team at Neo Matrix Medical consists of licensed MD's, DO's, ARNP's and Registered Sonographers. In addition, all our Health Care Professionals are Certified and Trained in the specific procedures we provide.

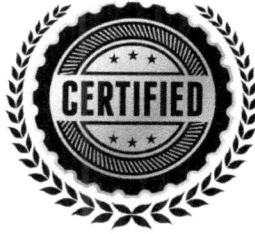

At Neo Matrix Medical, we ONLY PROVIDE REGENERATIVE MEDICINE treatments and services. We specialize in these Regenerative Medicine procedures.

At Neo Matrix Medical, we ONLY treat conditions shown to be effective according to Scientific Evidence.

At Neo Matrix Medical, we have performed 1000's of procedures over the past 4 years.

We use an FDA approved lab for our products and have strategically partnered with the Team at BioStem Technologies, allowing us to have the most innovative and up-to-date protocols to treat outpatients.

At Neo Matrix Medical, we have a 24/7 legal team to our availability and obtain the advice of FDA consultants on a regular basis.

We are also members of the American Academy of Stem Cell Physicians:

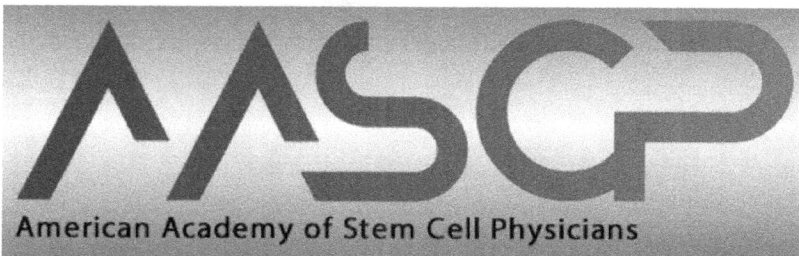

This allows us to stay at the forefront of the latest innovations and technologies in the field of Regenerative Medicine.

PRO-ATHLETES:

As a result of our VAST EXPERIENCE and most INNOVATIVE approach in Regenerative Medicine, we are proud to have PRO-ATHLETES, HALL OF FAMERS and WORLD CHAMPIONS and RECORD HOLDERS among our patients.

Most of these athletes do not allow us to use their names. But here are a few that did:

Pinklon Thomas "PINK", 2 times Heavyweight WORLD CHAMPION Boxing

In the pictures below with Evander Holyfield, on the left in 1988 at Caesars Palace in Las Vegas, and on the right in April of 2019 in Orlando.

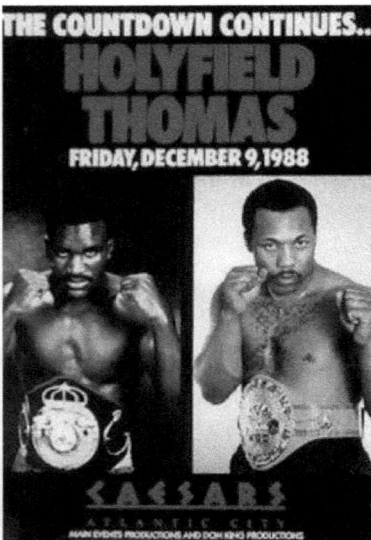

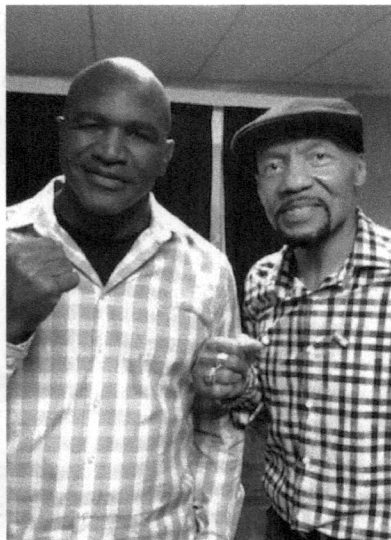

Pink was treated at our offices with the NEO SYNERGY protocol for his lower back and his left knee.

Ron Dixon, Former NFL Star / NY GIANTS

Most notable performance:

97-yard kick return for a touchdown in Super Bowl XXXV.

He also recorded a 97-yard kickoff return for a touchdown in the Giants win over the Philadelphia Eagles in the Divisional playoffs that year.

Ron Dixon has the Record for the most kickoff returns for a touchdown in a postseason campaign.

After some "stem cell type" (adipose) treatments a few years earlier that did not work for Ron, he was treated successfully at our offices with the NEO SYNERGY protocol for both knees.

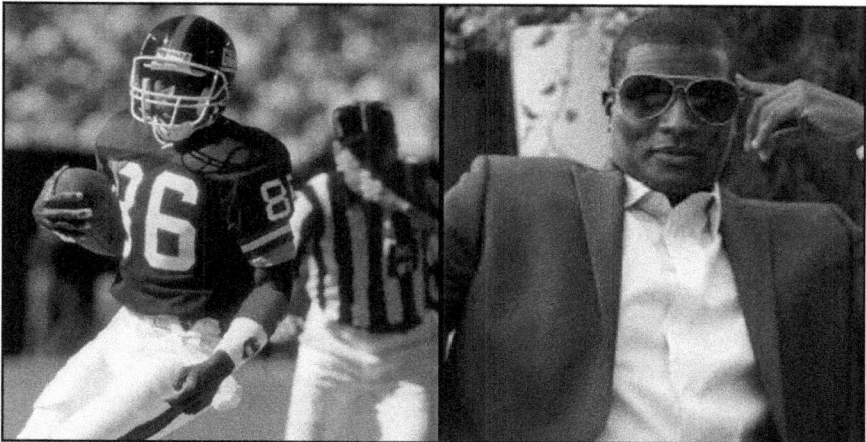

Curtis Mitchell or also known as Mr. 200

Curtis was 3rd at the 2013 World Championships, behind Usain Bolt.

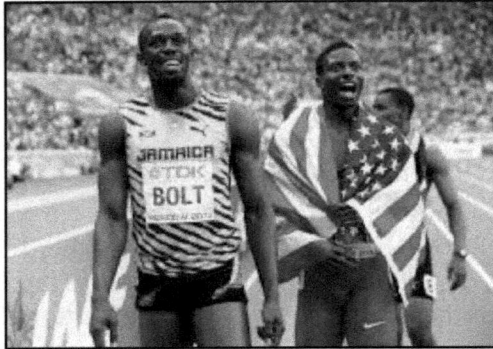

In 2014: Curtis became the American National champion in 200 meters in Sacramento, California. Curtis ranked number 1 in the world two consecutive years: 2013 and 2014

Currently, Curtis is training hard and going for GOLD TOKYO 2020

Mr. 200 was treated successfully at our offices with the NEO SYNERGY protocol for Achilles tendonitis, plantar fasciitis and a shoulder injury.

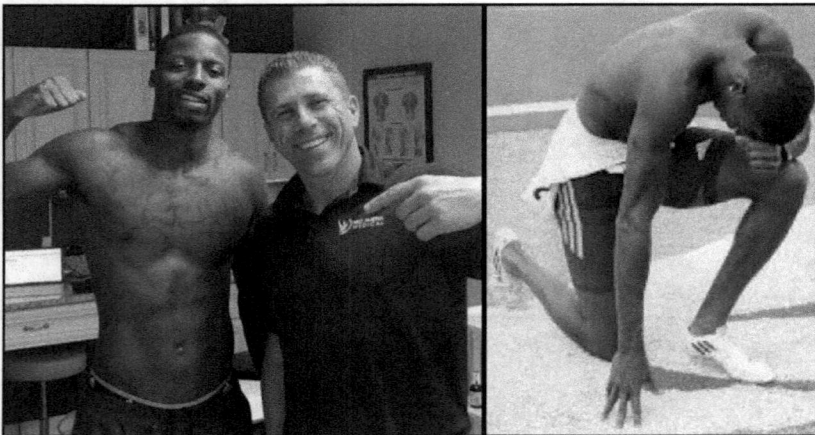

Conclusion:

EXPERIENCE is important. The Medical Team at Neo Matrix Medical has a vast experience in these specific Regenerative Medicine treatment modalities and has all the resources available to provide its patients and pro-athletes with the most innovative and up-to-date applications.

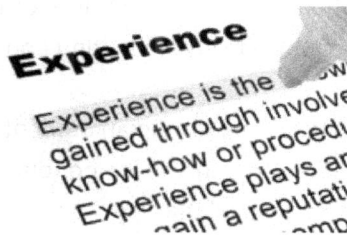

QUESTION 6: DO THEY OPERATE WITHIN THE POLICIES RECOMMENDED BY THE FSMB (FEDERATION OF STATE MEDICAL BOARDS)?

This policy protects the patient from a growing number of providers and clinics undermining the field of regenerative medicine. Such providers and clinics have been known to apply, prescribe or recommend stem cell-based therapies inappropriately, over-promise without sufficient data to support claims, and exploit patients who are often in desperate circumstances and willing to try any proposed therapy as a last resort, even if there is excessive or scant evidence of efficacy.

At Neo Matrix Medical, we proactively protect ourselves and

prospective patients by incorporating the following actions:

- We use an informed and shared decision-making process
- We discuss the benefits and risks of the treatment accurately, based on scientific evidence.
- We explain alternatives to the treatment
- We explain the right to withdraw from the treatment without denial of the standard of care to the patient
- We give the patient an opportunity to express preferences and values before collaboratively evaluating and arriving at treatment decisions
- We identify physician and physician credentials
- We determine if the diagnosis or condition is appropriate for regenerative and stem cell therapy
- We try to avoid to over-emphasize, exaggerate, inflate or misrepresent information provided verbally or in print.
- We try to avoid claims that are deceptive and present information based on scientific evidence
- We do not take advantage of patients that are desperate
- We don't treat conditions that are not proven effective
- We only treat conditions with regenerative and stem cell therapy when traditional or accepted proven treatment modalities have been exhausted
- We do not charge excessive fees for our treatment
- We practice within FDA guidelines and recommendations

Conclusion:

The Neo Matrix Medical Team is a proponent and advocate of the Policy set forth by the Federation of State Medical Boards. We have adopted this policy and incorporated it's guidelines and recommendations to protect the patient.

QUESTION 7: HOW ARE THE RESULTS QUANTIFIED WITH THEIR PATIENTS?

The Medical Team's at Neo Matrix Medical / Vitality Health have performed thousands of procedures over the past 4 years. At Neo Matrix Medical, we specialize in Regenerative Medicine, including allograft injections and SoftWave Therapy.

We treat patients with conditions that recent literature and published research, along with our vast experience, show to be responding very well to our pure product. These conditions include orthopedic conditions, sports injuries, eye conditions, chronic wounds, diabetic ulcers and E.D. (erectile dysfunction).

There are no guarantees in medicine, period. However, our current success rate across our clinics nationwide is EXCELLENT. We contribute our high success rate to:

- SUPERIOR PRODUCT - SAFE

- FDA APPROVED LAB (ISO 5)

- DIAGNOSTIC MSK ULTRASOUND

- SOFTWAVE THERAPY

- EXPERIENCED TEAM

- ONLY TREAT CONDITIONS PROVEN EFFECTIVE

- TRACK PROGRESS SCIENTIFICALLY

Just a few of our many before and after imaging results of our own patients:

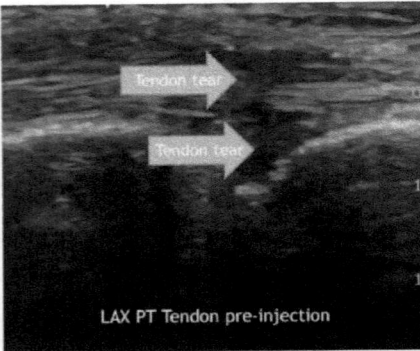

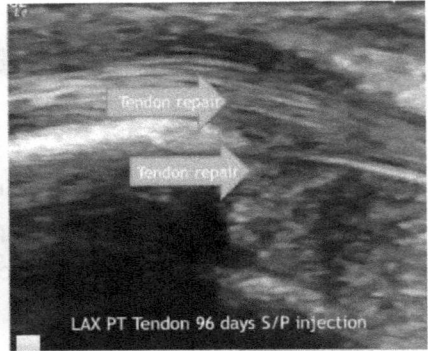

On the images above, we see a before and after of one of our patients. On the left we can see the posterior tibial tendon of the right ankle, revealing a tear as represented by the dark or black area. On the right image, you can visualize the same tendon 96 days after product placement, revealing a complete remodeling and regeneration of the tendon.

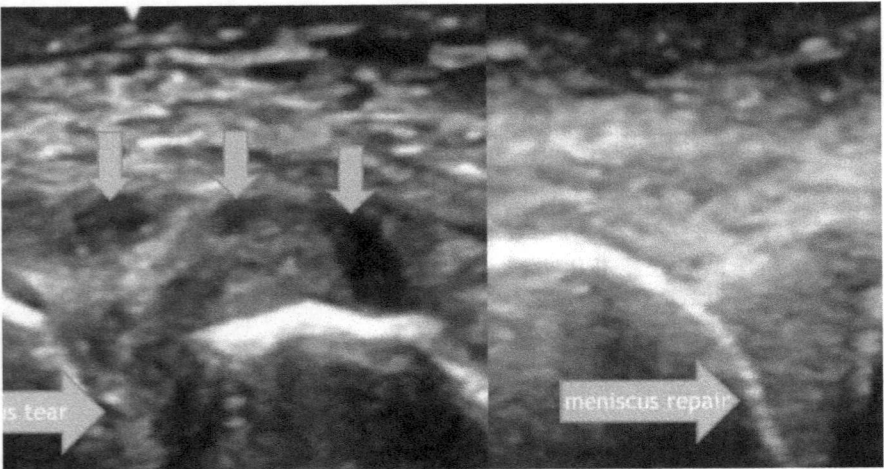

On the images above, we can see the medial meniscus and MCL of a patient who had injured his knee playing Frisbee on the beach. On the left, you can clearly see the multiple dark areas representing tears in the MCL. The medial meniscus, located in between the two bright lines (which represent bone) is also torn. On the right, we see an 81-day post-treatment image showing repair and regeneration of both the MCL and meniscus tears.

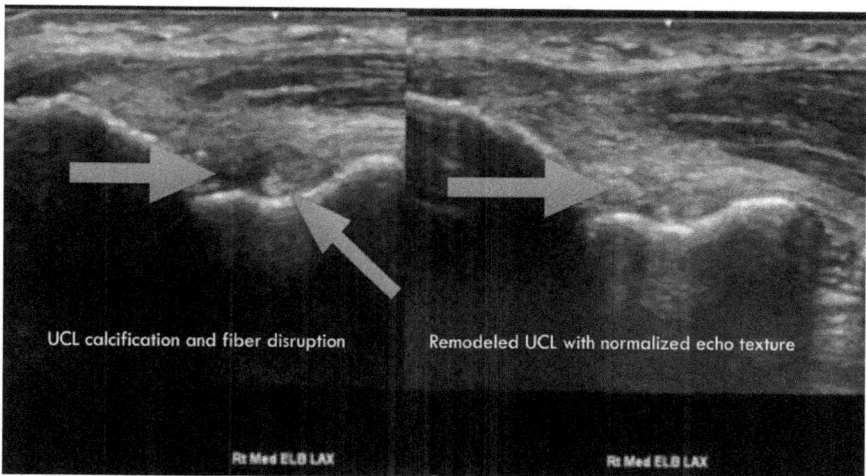

UCL calcification and fiber disruption   Remodeled UCL with normalized echo texture

Rt Med ELB LAX   Rt Med ELB LAX

On the images above (left), we can witness an ulnar collateral ligament (UCL) tear (or Tommy John injury). The patient is a male at age 50. He is an MD and works in the emergency room (ER) in a local hospital. He injured the medial aspect of his elbow many years ago while working out in the gym. The usual approach to this injury is a Tommy John reconstruction surgery in which the UCL is replaced with a tendon taken from elsewhere in the patient's body. Our patient stated that the success rate of this surgery, often performed on baseball pitchers and other athletes, is not great. That's why he decided to try the allograft injections. Within 3 months after the treatment, the patient reported zero pain and a significant increase in stability and strength of the elbow. He also reported he was able to push as much weight in the gym as when he was in college. On the right image, we can observe a complete repair of the UCL ligament.

We track our patient's progress carefully and objectively with Outcome MD.

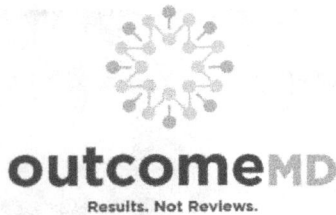

outcomeMD

Results. Not Reviews.

Outcome MD is an OBJECTIVE EVALUATION Tool that TRACKS & DEFINE IMPROVEMENT. Outcome MD employs the same type of questions used to establish a baseline and follow results for FDA studies and clinical trials.

Outcome MD is HIPAA compliant and secure.

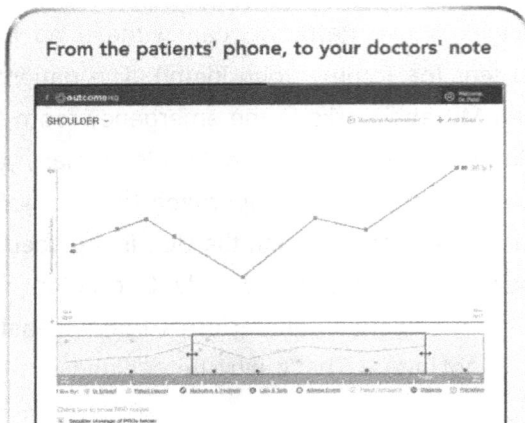

From the patients' phone, to your doctors' note

Conclusion:

At Neo Matrix Medical, we contribute our good results to our highly professional approach and vast experience.

CHAPTER 3

CONDITIONS TREATED

At Neo Matrix medical, we only treat conditions proven to be effective by scientific literature. These include:

- Sports Injuries
- Neuropathy
- Eye Conditions
- Chronic Wounds and Burns
- Diabetic Ulcers
- E.D. (Erectile Dysfunction)

A vast body of scientific research and trials has been conducted on many other medical conditions, such as MS, Parkinson's, RA, heart failure and respiratory disorders, diabetes, lupus, Alzheimer's, cancer, spinal cord injuries, autism, muscular dystrophy, ulcerative colitis, frailty in the elderly, and more. The treatment of these conditions in the U.S. is considered "off-label."

ORTHOPEDIC CONDITIONS

A vast body of scientific research and trials has been conducted on many other medical conditions, such as MS, Parkinson's, RA, heart failure and respiratory disorders, diabetes, lupus, Alzheimer's, cancer, spinal cord injuries,

Conventional approaches to arthritis and orthopedic conditions include prescription drugs, steroid injections, surgeries and physical therapy.

The prescription drugs may manage the symptoms of the condition but fail to repair the damaged tissues and address the underlying cause of the injury.

Steroid or cortisone injections may give the patient substantial relief by reducing the local inflammation of the injured area. However, it is no secret that steroids accelerate the deterioration of the joint. Quite frankly, these types of injections are a perfect set-up for replacement surgery.

Surgeries come with risks and often lack the desired results. These should be your last resort.

Scientific literature shows that the allograft injections with young

MSCs may help in the repair of many orthopedic and arthritic conditions:

Arthritis of small and large joints: knee, hip, shoulder, elbow, wrist/hands, ankles/feet, neck and back, TMJ, etc.

Spinal conditions: neck, mid-back and low back pain, spinal stenosis, degenerative conditions of the spine, arthritis of the spine, DDD, DJD, radiculopathies, sciatica, piriformis syndrome, SIJ dysfunction, etc.

Cartilage damage: osteoarthritis, cartilage degeneration, meniscus tears, arthritis, etc.

Tendon and bursa issues: tendon tears, rotator cuff tears, tendonitis, tenosynovitis, bursitis, etc.

Ligaments: Ligament tears (MCL, LCL, etc.) and sprains/strains

Muscles and soft tissue injuries: muscle tears, sprain and strains and all kinds of soft tissue injuries

Post-surgery & Scar management: post-operative healing and scar management, pain and damage post joint replacement or spinal surgery.

Other: Fractures, osteopenia and osteoporosis.

Sports Injuries

Acute and chronic sport-related injuries respond very well to stem cell therapies. At Neo Matrix Medical, we have successfully treated many athletes, including professional NFL players and world-class swimmers.

Benefits: avoiding surgery or invasive procedures, drastically reducing recovery or downtime, avoiding unnecessary adverse reactions, preventing further injuries and re-injury, prolonging professional career, repairing damaged tissue and engineering new and stronger tissue.

For more information, refer to "The Best Kept Secret in Professional Sports" below (page xx).

NEUROPATHY

Recent scientific literature shows that these young MSCs may help in the repair of small diameter nerve fibers as seen in peripheral neuropathy. Just one treatment can help to reestablish the local blood flow through the regeneration of the capillaries, which in turn helps with the regeneration of the small nerve fibers.

What is Neuropathy?

All of us, from the elbows down into the hands and from the knees down into the feet, have what we call: small diameter nerve fibers. In neuropathy patients, these small diameter nerve fibers are being killed off. Therefore, the neuropathy patient loses more and more of these small diameter nerve fibers. This results in a decrease in capillary volume, causing more pain, burning, numbness, inflammation and other symptoms.

However, the patient's balance also may be affected. In normal circumstances, the small diameter nerve fibers give constant feedback to the brain so we can walk without having to look at the ground and stay in balance. This is called proprioception. But when the patient loses more and more of these small diameter nerve fibers, balance and gait will be affected. The patient usually ends up having to use a cane or a walker to prevent falls.

How does this happen?

All of us have a brain, and the spinal cord is nothing but an extension of the brain. At each level of the spinal cord, large diameter nerve fibers come to exit the spinal canal to supply that particular area of the body. These large diameter nerve fibers are protected. They are protected by a myelin sheath, just as a wire that's insolated. However, the small diameter nerve fibers in our extremities do not have that protection, and that's where the neuropathy attacks.

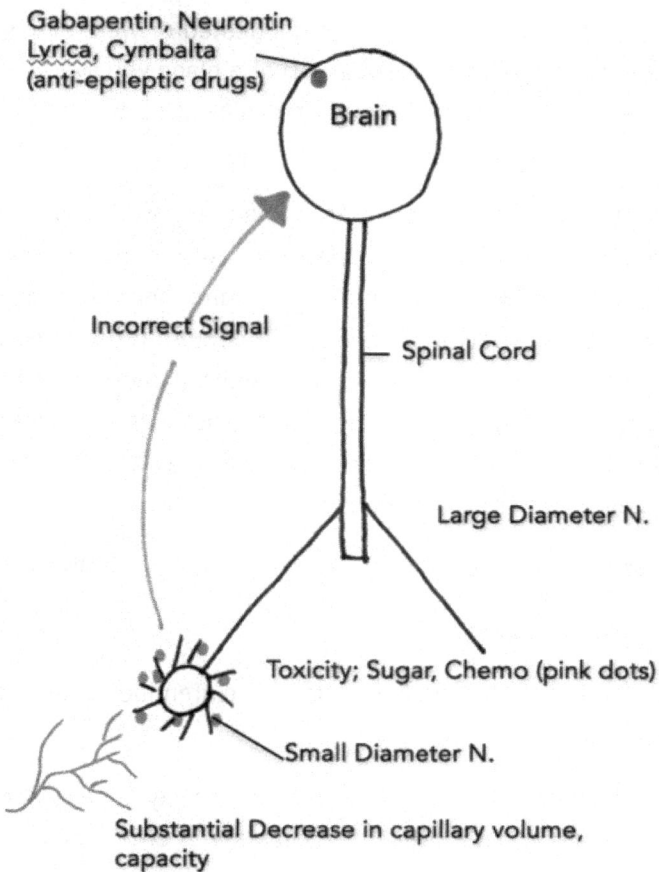

There are about a hundred causes of neuropathy. We all know of one: diabetes. But most patients are diagnosed with idiopathic neuropathy, meaning the cause is unknown. What we do know is that these unknown causes are toxins or toxicities. There are two good examples. When we look at our veterans, many of them suffer from neuropathy because they were exposed to agent orange. Many people who battled cancer and received strong chemotherapy (toxin) treatments often end up with neuropathy also. If you are not a veteran or a cancer patient, that simply means that during your lifetime you either ingested or were exposed to some type of toxin, maybe at a previous job or a place you lived (nobody knows). What we do know is that this toxin is slowly killing off more and more of those small diameter nerve fibers.

Conventional medicine has no solutions for neuropathy. Doctors usually prescribe medications such as Gabapentin, Neurontin, Lyrica and Cymbalta. These drugs are anti-epileptic drugs and therefore prescribed off-label for neuropathy patients. So why are doctors prescribing these drugs then? Because they have no solution and they hope these drugs reduce the pain levels of the neuropathy. I have to admit that a fair amount of neuropathy patients experience less pain when taking these drugs, however, the neuropathy simply continues to progress.

What would we have to accomplish to treat neuropathy effectively?

Two things would need to happen:

1. The blood flow or circulation in the extremities needs to be reestablished, and

2. As soon as the circulation returns, bringing oxygen and nutrients to the tissues and removing toxic substances and waste products

from the tissues, the small diameter nerve fibers can repair and regenerate.

In the image below, you can observe the four tissue biopsies of a neuropathy patient. The images show a gradual regeneration of new capillaries in the lower extremities of this patient.

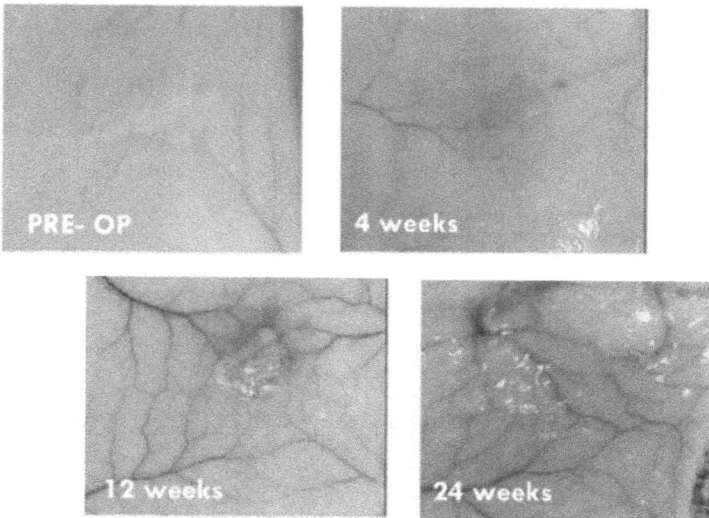

Regeneration of capillaries in Neuropathy

In the first picture, we can observe that many of the neuropathy patient's capillaries are dried up. It looks like a dried-up riverbed. This is typical for a neuropathy patient.

Four weeks after the allograft injection with young MSCs, we can notice a slow return of the capillaries.

Twelve weeks post treatment, we can see a significant increase in capillary volume and capacity, and at 24 weeks blood flow is back to normal.

During this process of capillary regeneration, the neuropathy patient will experience a gradual decrease in symptoms and a gradual improvement in balance and gait.

Scientific literature shows that the young MSCs effectively reverse the degeneration of nerves via the upregulation of NGF, NF-200 and angiogenesis.

At the end-stages of neuropathy, diabetic ulcers and osteomyelitis are common. These conditions may effectively be treated with the allograft membranes. Please review the section below: chronic wounds and diabetic ulcers.

EYE CONDITIONS

Scientific literature shows that these allograft membranes may help in the repair of many eye-related conditions such as dryness of the eyes and dry macular degeneration.

Dry eye disease (DED)

DED is one of the most common ocular surface disorders in the USA and worldwide. It affects nearly 30% of the population, and its symptoms, such as ocular discomfort and visual fluctuations, represent the most frequent complaints in ophthalmic practice.

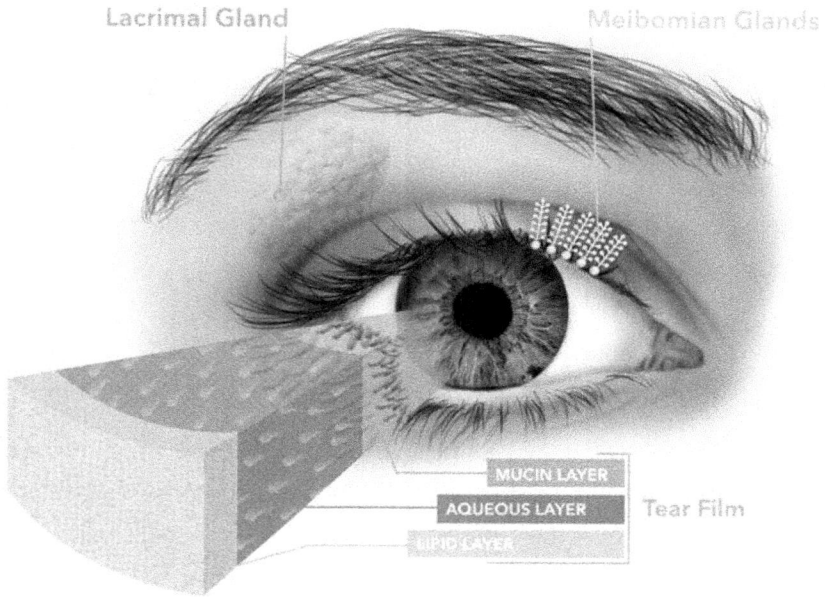

Lacrimal Gland   Meibomian Glands

MUCIN LAYER
AQUEOUS LAYER   Tear Film
LIPID LAYER

DED is comprised of tear film insufficiency and ocular surface involvement. Despite different underlying pathogenic processes, inflammation is a common denominator in DED, which in turn induces further damage to the corneal epithelium and its underlying structures.

Various treatment modalities, such as steroids and cyclosporine, have been used to suppress inflammation. However, results are variable and refractory in some cases. In these cases, DED not only negatively impacts the quality of life, but also increases the burden on health economics.

We use and Amnionic Membrane to treat eye conditions:

- The amniotic membrane reduces pain at the site of application.

- Amniotic membrane is non-immunogenic, has antibacterial properties, reduces inflammation and scar tissue. NO HLA markers / NO risk.

- The growth factors accelerate healing by stimulating angiogenesis and granulation tissue formation.

- Placental allografts are a pure product, carefully prepared for maximum effect and safety. No adverse events have been reported during its years of research, development and use.

At Neo Matrix Medical offices, we use the Vendaje OPTIC™ product:

- Vendaje OPTIC™ acts as a physical barrier to protect conjunctival and corneal epithelium as it heals, and it reduces pain caused by friction of the eyelids over the surface.

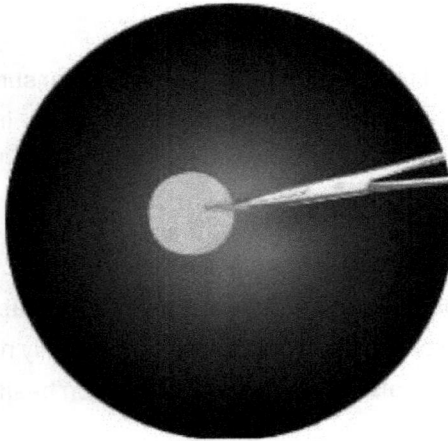

- The stroma of Vendaje OPTIC™, which contains fetal hyaluronic acid, inhibits fibroblast growth and reduces inflammation through decreased expression of cytokines.

- Vendaje OPTIC™ is applied directly to the eye and requires no surgical incisions for treatment.

- The amniotic membrane dissolves over one week, though it can last longer depending upon the clinical condition.

CHRONIC WOUNDS, BURNS and DIABETIC ULCERS

The annual cost of treating chronic wounds in the US is $25 Billion. Skin/ Dermal Substitutes is the largest segment of the chronic wound care market at $681 Million and sales of Placenta-Derived / Amniotic Tissue Products grew 33% to $305 Million (2017).

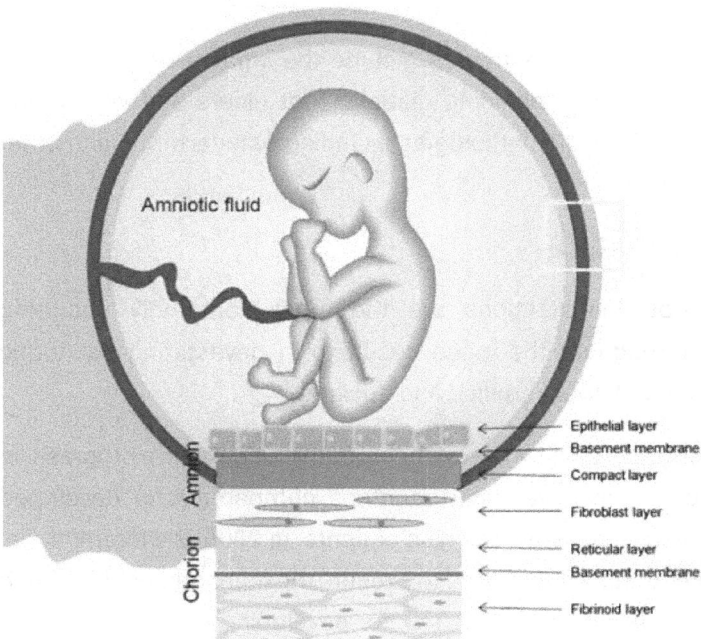

Amniotic fluid

Amnion

Chorion

Epithelial layer
Basement membrane
Compact layer
Fibroblast layer
Reticular layer
Basement membrane
Fibrinoid layer

Benefits of Amnionic Membrane application:

- The amniotic membrane reduces pain at the site of application, reducing or removing the need for traditional pain medication such as opioids.

- Amniotic membrane is non-immunogenic, has antibacterial properties, reduces inflammation and scar tissue.

- The growth factors accelerate healing by stimulating angiogenesis and granulation tissue formation.

- Placental allografts are a pure product, carefully prepared for maximum effect and safety. No adverse events have been reported during its years of research, development and use.

- Amniotic membrane treatments include the closing of chronic and non-healing wounds (including diabetic foot ulcers and venous leg ulcers) and orthopedic pathologies including osteoarthritis and other joint related issues.

Diabetic Foot Ulcers (DFU):

- Diabetic foot complications are the most commonly occurring problems throughout the globe, resulting in devastating economic crises for the patients, families and society.

- Diabetic foot ulcers (DFUs) have a neuropathic origin with a progressive prevalence rate in developing countries compared with developed countries among diabetes mellitus patients. In 2005, the International Diabetes Federation committed to execute the management approach for diabetic foot diseases. The risk for developing foot ulcers is 25% higher in patients with diabetes and it is also reported that every 30 seconds, one lower limb amputation in diabetes patients occurred around the world. A previously published study showed that the average annual expenditure of diabetic foot care is US$8659 per patient.

Diabetic Foot Ulcer

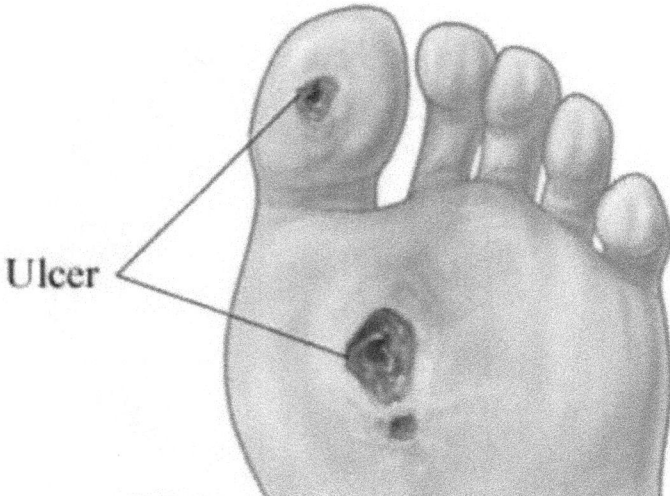

Ulcer

- The total medical cost for the management of diabetic foot disease in the United States (US) ranges from US$9 to US$13 billion in addition to the cost for management of DM alone. It is estimated in diabetic patients that of all amputations, 85% are contributed by foot ulceration, which further deteriorates to chronic infection and severe forms of gangrene.

At Neo Matrix Medical offices, we use Vendaje™ for chronic wounds and diabetic ulcers:

- Vendaje™ bonds with wounds by forming fibrin-elastin at the wound-dressing interface. This ensures excellent wound adherence and creates a moist environment that protects exposed nerve endings from irritants, providing pain relief, and creating an ideal environment for the regeneration at the surface of the wound.

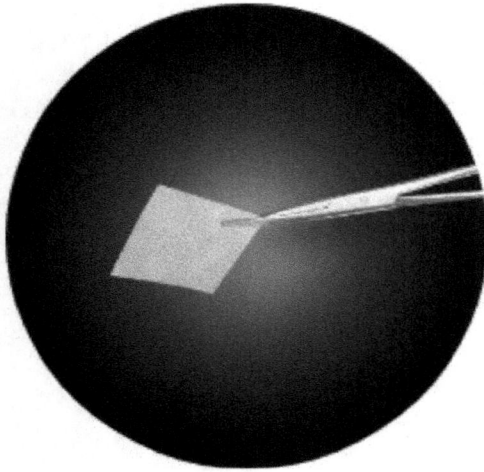

- In addition, the amnion layers make an excellent vapor barrier, preventing fluid loss from excessive evaporation from the wound surface.

- The associated factors in the membrane matrix also promote angiogenesis and neovascularization, which further promotes healing.

- Designed for application directly to acute and chronic wounds.

- Reduces scarring by supporting wound closure without excessive fibrosis.

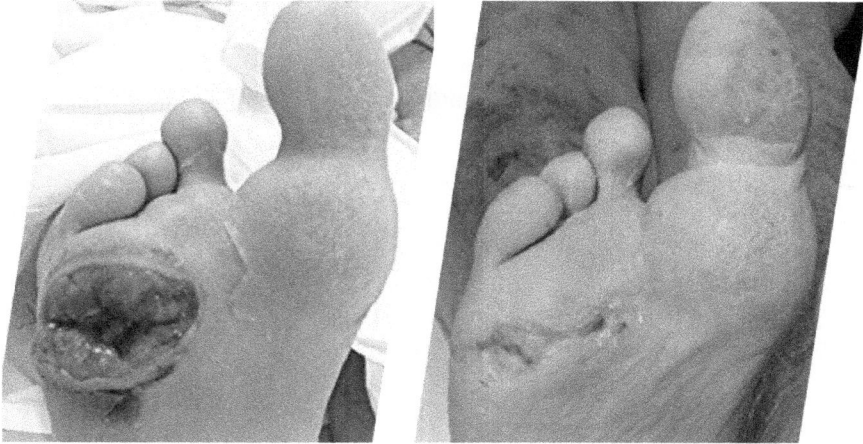

Diabetic Foot Ulcer (DFU) before the application of the Amnionic Membrane (left) and 9 weeks after (right).

E.D. (ERECTILE DYSFUNCTION)

Scientific literature shows that these tissue allografts with young MSCs and SoftWave therapy may help in the repair of the damaged penile tissue and can restore proper function.

E.D. can be caused by medications, surgeries, smoking, drinking, diabetes, heart disease, stress and depression, and relationship problems, among others.

These result in:

1. Poor Blood flow and microcirculation, which in turn depletes the cavernosal tissue (reservoir).

2. Impaired scaffolding support of the reservoirs which results in trouble

71

maintaining an erection.

3. Impaired function and overuse due to bio-physiological stresses and aging.

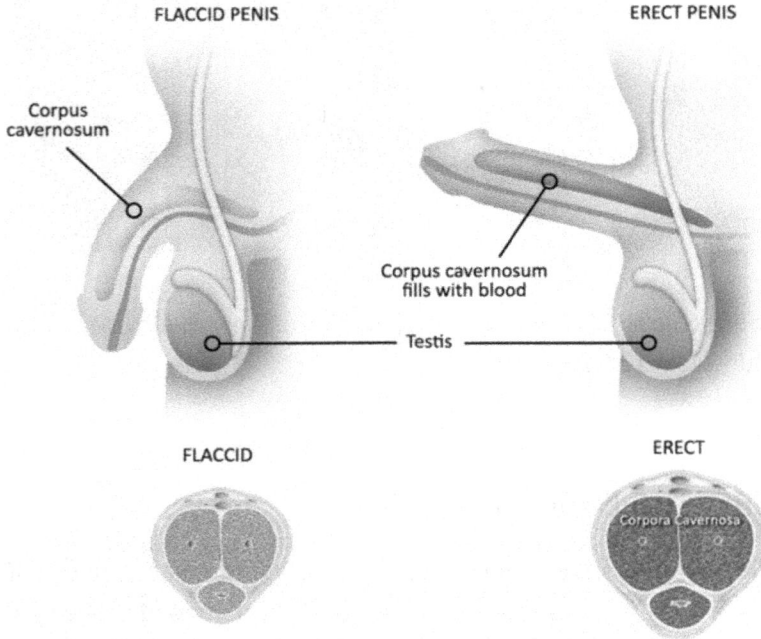

FLACCID PENIS

ERECT PENIS

Corpus cavernosum

Corpus cavernosum fills with blood

Testis

FLACCID

ERECT

Corpora Cavernosa

The conventional approaches to E.D. include:

1. PDE 5 inhibitors: Viagra, Cialis, Levitra

2. Genito-Urinary Prostaglandins: Muse (suppository)

3. Tri-mex & Bi-mex injections (at 3-day intervals)

The suppositories and injections are not the most consumer friendly and therefore, not very popular. Medications need to be taken daily.

Allograft injections and/or SoftWave therapy may restore blood flow, repair damaged tissue and address the fibrous plaque in Peyronie's Disease.

Peyronie's disease is defined as a bent or curvature of the penis due to a build-up of scar tissue.

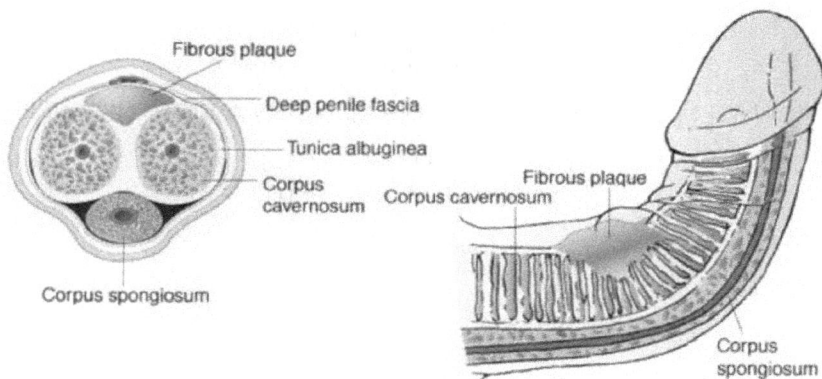

The conditions mentioned above are treated based on scientific research.

"Some groups criticize the stem cell industry by using the argument that if you're able to treat so many things with one 'drug' it must be snake oil or quackery. I'd like to address that here. Given that these cells are potently anti-inflammatory, able to modulate and even fix a broken immune system, and secrete molecules that stimulate regeneration, it only makes sense that they're able to treat conditions in which those particular processes are out of balance. For example, autism is really an inflammatory disease, as witnessed by elevated inflammatory markers. Autoimmune diseases are not only a dysfunctionality of the immune system, but upstream of that, also a dysfunctionality or depletion of the MSCs. In spinal cord injury, the problem is a lack of MSCs secreting molecules that stimulate regeneration. In these three very disparate conditions, the underlying mechanism is addressed by the MSCs. And that applies to almost every condition since there's not enough regeneration going on, too much inflammation, or a dysfunctional immune system."

STEM CELL THERAPY
A RISING TIDE
HOW STEM CELLS ARE DISRUPTING MEDICINE AND TRANSFORMING LIVES
Neil Riordan PA, PhD

CHAPTER 4

THE BEST KEPT SECRET IN PROFESSIONAL SPORTS

The best-kept secret in professional sports is becoming understood as the silver bullet in a team's armamentarium. Top Sports Medical clinicians across the world have been quietly using Allograft injections ("Stem Cell" therapies) and SoftWave therapy for years on their injured star athletes, seeing an unprecedented acceleration of recovery times. As success after success mounts, the Allograft and SoftWave synergy therapy is now becoming more widely understood to be the profound advantage that makes a tangible difference to who plays on the field and who stays in rehab.

Benefits for the PRO-ATHLETE and TEAM:

1. Avoiding surgery or invasive procedures

2. Significantly reducing recovery time or downtime

3. Avoiding unnecessary adverse reactions

4. Preventing further injuries and re-injury

5. Prolonging professional career

6. Repairing damaged tissue and re-engineering new and stronger tissue

7. Increased muscle mass and muscle strength, ROM and flexibility

8. No scarring

SPORTS INJURIES

Acute and chronic sport-related injuries respond very well to Allograft and SoftWave therapies. At Neo Matrix Medical, we have successfully treated many athletes, including professional NFL players and world-class boxers and swimmers.

Scientific literature shows that these therapies may help in the repair of many orthopedic and arthritic conditions:

Arthritis of small and large joints: knee, hip, shoulder, elbow, wrist/hands, ankles/feet, neck and back, TMJ, etc.

Spinal conditions: neck, mid-back and low back pain, spinal stenosis, degenerative conditions of the spine, arthritis of the spine, radiculopathies, sciatica, piriformis syndrome, SIJ dysfunction, etc.

Cartilage damage: osteoarthritis, cartilage degeneration, meniscus tears, arthritis, etc.

Tendon and bursa issues: tendon tears, rotator cuff tears, tendonitis, tendosynovitis, bursitis, plantar fasciitis, etc.

Ligaments: Ligament tears (MCL, LCL, etc.) and sprains/strains.

Muscles and soft tissue injuries: muscle tears, sprain and strains and all kinds of soft tissue injuries.

Post-surgery and Scar management: post-operative healing and scar management, pain and damage post joint replacement or spinal surgery.

INJURY PREVENTION and CAREER EXTENSION

At Neo Matrix Medical, we recommend treating the pro-athletes preventatively. Treating the joints and soft tissues that are most stressed with the specific athletic performance, heals and repairs the micro-traumas. Therefore, micro-trauma do not accumulate and eventually result in an injury.

This preventative approach prevents injury and lengthens the career of the athlete.

PERFORMANCE ENHANCEMENT

The allograft tissues not only repair damaged tissue but also renew and re-engineer this tissue to be new. New tissue is stronger, more flexible and more resilient.

Scientific literature also shows significant increases in muscle mass and muscle strength when these therapies are applied for that purpose.

PROFESSIONAL ATHLETES TREATED
(keep in mind that most pro-athletes do NOT allow us to use their names)

ALLOGRAFT INJECTIONS performed at our offices:

Ron Dixon, NFL superstar with NY Giants

Atlanta Falcons WR, Taylor Gabriel

Marlon Moore, WR (Dolphins, 49-ers, Browns)

2-time Heavyweight Champion of the World, Thomas Pinklon "Pink"

Curtis Mitchell, U.S. National Champion and medalist at the World Championships Track & Field, 200m in 2013

Mike Van Thielen, Master Swimming World Record holder and 21x U.S. National Master Champion

SOFTWAVE THERAPY recipients:

Tampa Bay Buccaneer RB, Ronald Jones, II

Former NFL Defensive Back and Sportscaster, Beasley Reece

Atlanta Falcons WR, Julian Williams

NFL Legend, Lawrence Tayler ("LT")

Former Philly Eagles WR and Athletes For Vets Founder, Dereck Faulkner

Ron Dixon, NFL superstar with NY Giants

Retired MLB Star, Atlee Hammaker

NY Yankees Minor League Player, Kellin Deglan

Curtis Mitchell, U.S. National Champion and medalist at the World Championships Track & Field, 200m in 2013.

Indoor Long Jump Champion and UF Grad, Marquis Dendy

Pro Heavyweight Boxer entity, Brandon "Bulletproof" Blanton

2-time Heavyweight Champion of the World, Thomas Pinklon "Pink"

Pro Rugby player, Jeremy Noble

Pro Tennis Player, Dean O'Brien

Mike Van Thielen, Master Swimming World Record holder and 21x U.S. National Master Champion

Medical Institutions & Pro Sports Teams utilizing SoftWave Therapy:

Cleveland Indians (Baseball)

Chicago Cubs (Baseball)

Synergy Sports Release in Alpharetta, GA

Shepherd Spine Center, Atlanta, GA

For an incomplete list of Top Athletes around the world who received stem cell-based therapies, please refer to ADDENDUM 3.

At Neo Matrix Medical, we use the most innovative HCT/P (Human

CHAPTER 5

REALISTIC EXPECTATIONS

The allografts from birth tissue are SAFE and do not cause any adverse reactions. No blood typing is necessary. No rejection is possible, and no allergic reactions have been reported. Only an allergic reaction to the preservatives (DMSO) is possible.

There are NO drugs involved in these procedures, and there's No surgery needed to harvest MSCs either.

There is NO downtime and usually, ONLY 1 treatment is required to obtain the desired results.

MSCs have a strong anti-inflammatory effect. Therefore, many patients experience some relief within a few days or weeks of the treatment. That doesn't mean the MSCs have already repaired and renewed the injured cells or tissues. The relief is because of the anti-inflammatory properties.

The full benefit of allograft application is usually obtained in 3-6 months post-treatment. So, patience is the key. The tissue did not degenerate overnight and it takes some time to repair and renew.

SUMMARY

When researching 'stem cells' or when considering 'stem cell therapy', one has to be careful with his/her provider selection since not all allograft products contain all essential components for tissue engineering. Also, not all manufacturers are compliant with current FDA regulations, and not all providers adopt the policy set forth by the Federation of State Medical Boards to protect the patient. Be aware that some providers take advantage of patients that may be desperate.

Cellular Tissue or Product) to treat our patients. Most providers use products that are missing essential components for effective tissue repair and engineering. The essential components for tissue engineering include MSCs (Medicinal Signaling Cells), growth factors, cytokines, collagens, exosomes, and scaffolding (ECM).

Be aware that many providers and manufacturers alike market and compete by comparing the number of live MSC's in their product. This is irrelevant because even cells in apoptosis can release bio-active molecules in the recipient.

For better and faster results, MSK Ultrasound imaging is used to safely diagnose and accurately place the product in the injured areas. Unlike with so-called "blind" injections (absence of an imaging modality), accurate placement allows for optimal results.

The addition of SoftWave Therapy allows for a synergistic approach, called NEO SYNERGY, and significantly improves patient outcomes.

At Neo Matrix Medical / Vitality Health, we have performed thousands of Regenerative Medicine procedures over the past 4 years and we have an excellent success rate for the conditions that we treat. We contribute our success to our highly professional approach and vast experience.

ADDENDUM 1

FDA Nov. 2020 NOTICE

The FDA regulates "stem cell" products to treat a variety of diseases or conditions under the Public Health Service Act (PHS Act) as human cells, tissues, or cellular or tissue-based products (HCT/Ps), as defined in 21 CFR 1271.3 (d). Although generally regulated as HCT/Ps, such products may also be regulated under the PHS Act and the Federal Food, Drug, and Cosmetic Act (FD&C Act), as biological products, drugs, and/or devices, and may require pre-market review.

FDA's November 2017 comprehensive regenerative medicine policy framework is intended to spur innovation and efficient access to safe and effective regenerative medicine products, including HCT/Ps.

FDA's final guidance, Regulatory Considerations for Human Cell, Tissues, and Cellular and Tissue-Based Products: Minimal Manipulation and Homologous Use, issued November 2017 (copy attached), informed manufacturers, health care providers, and other interested parties about the Agency's compliant and enforcement policy for these products. The guidance outlines the FDA's intent to exercise enforcement discretion for the first 36 months following the issuance of the guidance for certain products with respect to FDA's IND (Investigational New Drug) and premarket approval requirements when the product does not raise reported safety concerns or potential significant safety concerns. This period (until November of 2020) provides manufacturers time to comply with the IND and premarket approval requirements and engage with the FDA to determine whether they need to submit an IND or marketing authorization application and if so, to submit their application to the FDA.

The FDA is currently applying a risk-based approach to enforcement, accounting for how products are being administered and the diseases and conditions for which they are being used, in addition, the document states that the 36-month period during which FDA intends to exercise enforcement discretion will end November 2020.

Our Interpretation:

The Impact on the Industry, specific to Manufacturing

1. Manufacturers need to engage with the FDA to determine whether they need to submit an IND or marketing authorization application and if so, to submit their application to FDA, prior to November 2020.

2. The HCT/Ps currently regulated under Section 361 of 21 CFR 1271 (homologous use) eventually will need to be regulated under Section 351 (specific indications). This may or may not affect the manufacturing standards of these HCT/Ps. This means that IND's / clinical trials will need to be done and show efficacy for the HCT/P in correlation to a specific indication or condition.

How does this affect Providers?

1. Providers need to be cautious in the manner they market these products. The products are currently only recommended for homologous use and do not have any specific indications.

   Homologous use: The FDA "generally considers an HCT/P to be for homologous use when it is used to repair, reconstruct, replace, or supplement:

DR. MIKE VAN THIELEN

Recipient cells or tissues that are identical (e.g., skin for skin) to the donor cells or tissues, and perform one or more of the same basic functions in the recipient as the cells or tissues performed in the donor; or Recipient cells or tissues that may not be identical to the donor's cells or tissues, but that perform one or more of the same basic functions in the recipient as the cells or tissues performed in the donor.

At Neo Matrix Medical, we only treat conditions that conform to these guidelines and have been proven beneficial according to scientific literature.

2. Providers need to be cautious on how these products are being administered to their patients, and the diseases and conditions they use these products for.

    At Neo Matrix Medical, we only treat conditions that have been proven beneficial according to scientific literature. We administer our HCT/Ps peri-or intra-articular or IM (intra-muscular). We do not administer these products IV (intravenous).

3. Providers are reminded that the 36-month period during which the FDA intends to exercise enforcement discretion will end November 2020.

    At Neo Matrix Medical, we have engaged with the FDA directly. We adhere to the recommendations set forth and have acquired the services of FDA consultants.

    We continue to stay a few steps ahead and operate within the proposed framework, including the marketing, administration and treatment of conditions with these HCT/Ps.

We have aligned ourselves with BioStem Technologies, Inc. as our HCT/P manufacturer. BioStem Technolgies, Inc. has a state-of-the-art, FDA approved, certified ISO 5 laboratory. The safety measurements taken at BioStem Technologies exceed the FDA requirements.

Furthermore, BioStem Technologies, Inc. is actively in the process of submitting 4 IND's with the FDA.

BioStem Technologies, Inc. is taking the appropriate steps to be compliant by November 2020 and Neo Matrix Medical will be able to partake in the IND studies.

ADDENDUM 2

FDA WARNING AND OUR RESPONSE

FDA Warns About Stem Cell Therapies

Stem cells have been called everything from cure-alls to miracle treatments. But don't believe the hype. Some unscrupulous providers offer stem cell products that are both unapproved and unproven. So beware of potentially dangerous procedures—and confirm what's really being offered before you consider any treatment.

The facts: Stem cell therapies may offer the potential to treat diseases or conditions for which few treatments exist. Sometimes called the body's "master cells," stem cells are the cells that develop into blood, brain, bones, and all of the body's organs. They have the potential to repair, restore, replace, and regenerate cells, and could possibly be used to treat many medical conditions and diseases.

But the U.S. Food and Drug Administration is concerned that some patients seeking cures and remedies are vulnerable to stem cell treatments that are illegal and potentially harmful. And the FDA is increasing its oversight and enforcement to protect people from dishonest and unscrupulous stem cell clinics while continuing to encourage innovation so that the medical industry can properly harness the potential of stem cell products.

To do your part to stay safe, make sure that any stem cell treatment you are considering is either:

- FDA-approved, or;

- Being studied under an Investigational New Drug Application (IND), which is a clinical investigation plan submitted and allowed to proceed by the FDA.

And see the boxed section below for more advice.

Stem Cell Uses and FDA Regulation

The FDA has the authority to regulate stem cell products in the United States.

Today, doctors routinely use stem cells that come from bone marrow or blood in transplant procedures to treat patients with cancer and disorders of the blood and immune system.

With limited exceptions, investigational products must also go through a thorough FDA review process as investigators prepare to determine the safety and effectiveness of products in well-controlled human studies, called clinical trials. The FDA has reviewed many stem cell products for use in these studies.

As part of the FDA's review, investigators must show how each product will be manufactured so the FDA can make sure appropriate steps are being taken to help assure the product's safety, purity, and strength (potency). The FDA also requires sufficient data from animal studies to help evaluate any potential risks associated with product use. (You can learn more about clinical trials on the FDA's website.)

That said, some clinics may inappropriately advertise stem cell clinical trials without submitting an IND. Some clinics also may falsely advertise that FDA review and approval of the stem cell therapy is unnecessary. But when clinical trials are not conducted under an IND, it means that the

FDA has not reviewed the experimental therapy to help make sure it is reasonably safe. So be cautious about these treatments.

About FDA-approved products derived from stem cells

The only stem cell-based products that are FDA-approved for use in the United States consist of blood-forming stem cells (hematopoietic progenitor cells) derived from cord blood.

These products are approved for limited use in patients with disorders that affect the body system that is involved in the production of blood (called the "hematopoietic" system). These FDA-approved stem cell products are listed on the FDA website. Bone marrow also is used for these treatments but is generally not regulated by the FDA for this use.

Safety Concerns for Unproven Stem Cell Treatments

All medical treatments have benefits and risks. But unproven stem cell therapies can be particularly unsafe.

For instance, attendees at a 2016 FDA public workshop discussed several cases of severe adverse events. One patient became blind due to an injection of stem cells into the eye. Another patient received a spinal cord injection that caused the growth of a spinal tumor.

Other potential safety concerns for unproven treatments include:

- Administration site reactions,

- The ability of cells to move from placement sites and change into inappropriate cell types or multiply,

- Failure of cells to work as expected, and

- The growth of tumors.

Note: Even if stem cells are your own cells, there are still safety risks such as those noted above. In addition, if cells are manipulated after removal, there is a risk of contamination of the cells.

FDA Actions on Unapproved Stem Cell Products

When stem cell products are used in unapproved ways—or when they are processed in ways that are more than minimally manipulated, which relates to the nature and degree of processing—the FDA may take (and has already taken) a variety of administrative and judicial actions, including criminal enforcement, depending on the violations involved.

In August 2017, the FDA announced increased enforcement of regulations and oversight of stem cell clinics. To learn more, see the statement from FDA Commissioner Scott Gottlieb, M.D., on the FDA website.

And in March 2017, to further clarify the benefits and risks of stem cell therapy, the FDA published a perspective article in the New England Journal of MedicineExternal Link Disclaimer.

The FDA will continue to help with the development and licensing of new stem cell therapies where the scientific evidence supports the product's safety and effectiveness.

Advice for People Considering Stem Cell Therapies

Stem cell products have the potential to treat many medical conditions and diseases. But for almost all of these products, it is not yet known whether the product has any benefit—or if the product is safe to use.

If you're considering treatment in the United States:

- Ask if the FDA has reviewed the treatment. Ask your health care provider to confirm this information. You also can ask the clinical investigator to give you the FDA-issued Investigational New Drug Application number and the chance to review the FDA communication acknowledging the IND. Ask for this information before getting treatment—even if the stem cells are your own.

- Request the facts and ask questions if you don't understand. To participate in a clinical trial that requires an IND application, you must sign a consent form that explains the experimental procedure. The consent form also identifies the Institutional Review Board (IRB) that assures the protection of the rights and welfare of human subjects. Make sure you understand the entire process and known risks before you sign. You also can ask the study sponsor for the clinical investigator's brochure, which includes a short description of the product and information about its safety and effectiveness.

If you're considering treatment in another country:

- Learn about regulations that cover products in that country.

- Know that the FDA does not have oversight of treatments done in other countries. The FDA typically has little information about foreign establishments or their stem cell products.

- Be cautious. If you're considering a stem cell-based product in a country that may not require regulatory review of clinical studies, it may be hard to know if the experimental treatment is reasonably safe.

NEO MATRIX MEDICAL RESPONSE

Recently the FDA issued a warning to consumers regarding the use of stem cell therapies. We would like to take this opportunity to address their concerns and discuss the key takeaways from this warning.

The FDA warning letter reflects their concerns regarding "stem cell therapies", however, our clinic offers regenerative medicine therapies and we no longer use the language "stem cell therapy."

At Neo Matrix Medical, we understand that chronic painful conditions can render people desperate for help and vulnerable to unscrupulous clinics. This is a true concern for the consumer and one that we appreciate the FDA bringing to light.

That's why we operate within the policies recommended by the Federation of State Medical Boards (FSMB). This policy protects the patient from a growing number of providers and clinics undermining the field of regenerative medicine.

Such providers and clinics have been known to apply, prescribe or recommend stem cell-based therapies inappropriately, over-promise without sufficient data to support claims, and exploit patients who are often in desperate circumstances and willing to try any proposed therapy as a last resort, even if there is excessive or scant evidence of efficacy.

At Neo Matrix Medical, we proactively protect ourselves and prospective patients by incorporating the following actions:

- We use an informed and shared decision-making process.

- We discuss the benefits and risks of the treatment accurately, based on scientific evidence.

- We explain alternatives to the treatment.

- We explain the right to withdraw from the treatment without a denial of the standard of care to the patient.

- We give the patient an opportunity to express preferences and values before collaboratively evaluating and arriving at treatment decisions.

- We identify provider and provider credentials.

- We determine if the diagnosis or condition is appropriate for regenerative therapy.

- We try to avoid to over-emphasize, exaggerate, inflate or misrepresent information provided verbally or in print.

- We try to avoid claims that are deceptive and present information based on scientific evidence.

- We do not take advantage of patients that are desperate.

- We don't treat conditions that are not proven effective.

- We only treat conditions with regenerative and stem cell therapy when traditional or accepted proven treatment modalities have been exhausted.

- We do not charge excessive fees for our treatment.

- We practice within FDA guidelines and recommendations

Within the body of the warning, the FDA states "To do your part to stay safe, make sure that any stem cell treatment you are considering is either:

- FDA-approved, or;

- Being studied under an Investigational New Drug Application (IND), which is a clinical investigation plan submitted and allowed to proceed by the FDA."

As stated, currently, the FDA has only "approved" stem cell therapy for certain blood disorders. At Neo Matrix Medical, we focus on conditions that are currently involved in an IND. Those conditions are osteoarthritis (OA) and peripheral neuropathy and have been extensively researched in animal models, in vitro and in vivo. We work with tissue allografts that do not just focus on "mesenchymal stem cells (MSC's)" but rather focus on a broad array of components.

Remember that MSCs do NOT repair and heal damaged tissue, but rather the synergistic workings between all the essential components or bio-active molecules released in the environment that allow the body to repair, renew and reengineer tissues and cells.

We work with Rheo for tissue engineering, which has all essential components for tissue engineering:

- Amniotic Membrane (ECM: scaffolding and collagens)

- Amniotic fluid and Exosomes

- WJ (umbilical cord matrix): Young MSCs, cytokines, GFs

- Hyaluronic Acid (HA)

Please find two links below for IND's currently underway for the conditions we focus on.

IND for OA:

https://clinicaltrials.gov/ct2/show/
NCT03818737?term=osteoarthritis+AND +stem+cell&draw=4&rank=32

IND for Peripheral neuropathy

https://clinicaltrials.gov/ct2/show/NCT03899298?term=peripheral +neuropathy+AND+stem+cell&draw=3&rank=29

At Neo Matrix Medical, we take safety very seriously and work only with tissue allografts from FDA approved labs. These products are regulated by the FDA from procurement to the delivery to our clinic. We only work with products described and acknowledged by the FDA as "minimally manipulated." In fact, the tissue products we work with exceed FDA compliance. In addition, these tissues are known to be non-tumorigenic, meaning they CANNOT cause teratomas or tumors.

They have cited two very unfortunate examples of misuse and dangerous practices that have occurred in the field of regenerative medicine! We share their concerns in this matter and would never attempt such egregiously dangerous procedures.

It is important to note that the use of perinatal tissues has been ongoing for many years, with many thousands of procedures being performed. The FDA has highlighted two incidences but has failed to mention the many thousands of treatments in which no severe adverse reaction have occurred. FDA approval for treatment of these conditions with these tissues is very important and will occur over time. But FDA approval does not necessarily equate to safety as can be seen from this quote taken from Harvard University Center for Ethics, "few people know that new prescription drugs have a 1 in 5 chance of causing serious reactions after they have been approved. That is why expert physicians recommend not taking new drugs for at least five years unless patients have first tried better-established options, and have the need to do so.

Few know that systematic reviews of hospital charts found that even properly prescribed drugs (aside from mis-prescribing, overdosing, or self-prescribing) cause about 1.9 million hospitalizations a year. Another 840,000 hospitalized patients are given drugs that cause serious adverse reactions for a total of 2.74 million severe adverse drug reactions. About 128,000 people die from drugs prescribed to them. This makes prescription drugs a major health risk, ranking 4th with stroke as a leading cause of death. The European Commission estimates that adverse reactions from prescription drugs cause 200,000 deaths; so together, about 328,000 patients in the U.S. and Europe die from prescription drugs each year. The FDA does not acknowledge these facts and instead gathers a small fraction of the cases."

Currently, patients who are being treated for peripheral neuropathy are receiving treatment from their physicians that are off label and unapproved by the FDA. For example, Gabapentin is an anti-seizure medication that is routinely prescribed to neuropathy patients. This means there is no safety data or proof of efficacy for use in this way. The FDA appears to be okay with this practice." Link here. https://ethics.harvard.edu/blog/new-prescription-drugs-major-health-risk-few-offsetting-advantages

In our continued efforts to work in accordance with the FDA's guidance, we recently sent a certified letter to the FDA asking for additional information to help us remain compliant while operating in this dynamic field. As of the date of this writing, we have had no response yet from the FDA. We at Neo Matrix Medical will remain vigilant in our efforts to provide safe and efficacious treatment options to our patients that have exhausted all conventional options.

ADDENDUM 3

ALLOGRAFT INJECTIONS used by the WORLD's GREATEST ATHLETES

38 Pro Athletes Who Have Had Stem Cell Treatments

July 25, 2018, By Cade Hildreth (CEO Bioinformant.com)

More and more athletes are turning to stem cell treatments because the pressure to get back on the field is high and access to these regenerative medicine therapies is continuing to increase. Athletes commonly suffer serious injuries that could potentially end their careers and cause them serious long-term health complications. Most of them turn to surgery to resolve those injuries.

However, some of them are pursuing stem cell treatments because these procedures are less invasive than surgery and have the potential to speed and augment the repair.

Athletes and Their Stem Cell Treatments

This article outlines 38 athletes who have undergone stem cell treatments for their knees, hips, ankles, shoulders, and more.

In this article:

- Stem Cell Therapy for Knees

- ACL and MCL Stem Cell Therapy for Athletes

- Stem Cell Therapy for Cartilage, Tendon, & Muscles

- Elbow Stem Cell Treatments

- Leg and Foot Stem Cell Treatments

- Other Types of Stem Treatments for Athletes

- Stem Cell Treatments Beyond Injuries

- Stem Cell Therapy for Athletes

Stem Cell Therapy for Knees

The 14 athletes below pursed stem cell therapies to resolve knee injuries and complications.

1. Jarvis Green | Denver Broncos

In 2010, the NFL player Jarvis Green went to Regenexx to seek stem cell treatment for his knees. The treatment involved extracting stem cells from his bone marrow and then injecting it into his knees. Prior to this, Green had two knee surgeries, which both resulted in complications and long recovery periods.

2. Knowshon Moreno | Denver Broncos

The running back for the Denver Broncos also had stem cell treatment for his knees. He had his treatment in 2013 but has yet to disclose which stem cell clinic he used.

3. Sidney Rice | Seattle Seahawks

Sidney Rice went to Switzerland for stem cell injections. The Seattle Seahawks' wide receiver underwent Regenokine injection treatments for his knees.

4. Hines Ward | Pittsburgh Steelers

Hines Ward was among one of the first athletes who turned to stem cell treatment for a speedy recovery. He had joint regeneration therapy using cell prolotherapy at Intermountain Stem Cells. The treatment was for a knee medial collateral ligament sprain.

5. Adrian Clayborn | Atlanta Falcons

The defensive lineman for the Falcons underwent knee surgery and used stem cell therapy to speed up his recovery. The operation was for a torn medial collateral ligament in his left knee.

6. Jamaal Charles | Kansas City Chiefs

Jamaal Charles had a torn anterior cruciate ligament on his knee and had ligament-repair surgery. His stem cell therapy involved extracting stem cells from his bone marrow and injecting them into his knee.

7. Rolando McClain | Oakland Raiders

Rolando McClain had been experiencing chronic pain in his knees for two years, and then he suffered a high ankle sprain. During his offseason, McClain went to USA Precision Stem Cell and had liposuctioned fat cells autologously injected into his knees.

8. Aaron Curry | Oakland Raiders

The Raiders' linebacker injured both of his knees and then underwent stem cell treatment during his offseason.

9. Alex Rodriguez | New York Yankees

When Alex Rodriguez sustained a knee injury, he went to Germany for stem cell treatment. The procedure was a platelet-rich plasma therapy that was injected into Rodriguez's knee. They also injected it into his shoulder to prevent future inflammation.

10. Josh Hamilton | Texas Rangers

Josh Hamilton of the Texas Rangers had experienced swelling on his knee for a long time before he finally consulted with Dr. James Andrews to then received a stem cell and platelet-rich plasma injection.

11. Takashi Saito | L.A. Dodgers

The pitcher for the Los Angeles Dodgers didn't want to risk his career by allowing surgery on his knees. Instead, he went to joint Intermountain Stem Cells for regeneration therapy using stem cell prolotherapy.

12. Kobe Bryant | L.A. Lakers

Kobe Bryant traveled to Germany to seek stem cell treatment from Dr. Peter Wehling for the degeneration of his knees.

13. Pau Gasol | San Antonio Spurs

Pau Gasol had an autologous stem cell injection on his knee to remove degenerated tissue without surgery. The procedure was a focused aspiration scar tissue removal done by Dr. Steve Yoon at the Kerlan-Jobe Orthopaedic Clinic.

14. Chris Johnson | New York Jets

Chris Johnson sustained a meniscus injury on his left knee, but he continued to play through the season. The injury worsened, and Johnson lost a lot of cartilage throughout the remainder of the season. He sought out Dr. James Andrews and had stem cell therapy to accelerate his recovery.

ACL and MCL Stem Cell Therapy for Athletes

The three athletes below pursed stem cell therapies for ACL and MCL repair (ligaments within the human knee).

15. Tiger Woods | Professional Golfer

The famous golfer confirmed in 2010 that he had undergone a stem cell treatment. He received joint regeneration therapy with platelet-rich injections.

16. Stephen Curry | Golden State Warriors

Stephen Curry had a grade-1 MCL sprain and consulted with Dr. Russ Riggs from the Reflex Clinic in Tigard regarding stem cell treatments. Dr. Riggs advised Curry to have PRP injections to help his recovery by reducing the inflammation and pain.

17. Terrell Owens | Cincinnati Bengals

The former NFL player went to South Korea's Chaum Anti-Aging Center to seek treatment for an ACL injury. There, he had bone marrow-derived stem cell injections for ligaments, tendons, and joints.

Stem Cell Therapy for Cartilage, Tendon, & Muscles

The six athletes below pursed stem cell therapies to resolve cartilage, tendon, and muscle complications.

18. Uche Nwaneri | Jacksonville Jaguars

The Jacksonville Jaguars guard sought stem cell treatment for cartilage regrowth in 2013. However, Uche Nwaneri has not yet gone public about which clinic he underwent treatment.

19. Marquis Maze | Pittsburgh Steelers

Marquis Maze, the former University of Alabama receiver, had stem cell therapy for a muscle injury at USA Precision Stem Cell. The procedure was an autologous operation for his damaged joints and muscles.

20. LaRon Landry | Washington Redskins

LaRon Landry missed a lot of games in 2012 due to an injury to his left Achilles tendon. Instead of seeking surgery, he went to AminoMatrix and had PRP treatments for his torn tendon.

21. Cliff Lee | Philadelphia Phillies

Cliff Lee is one of the many athletes who has gone to Intermountain Stem Cells. According to their website, Lee had a joint regeneration therapy using stem cell prolotherapy.

22. Dara Torres | Olympic Swimmer

The Olympic swimmer had mild arthritis in her knees, which worsened due to her training. In 2009, she had autologous chondrocyte implantation to regrow the cartilage cells on her kneecap.

23. Israel Dagg | Crusaders

The veteran rugby player took a break from his career due to damaged knee cartilage. With the hope of reviving his career, he had stem cells injected into his right knee at a clinic in Queenstown.

Elbow Stem Cell Treatments

The three athletes below pursed stem cell therapies to resolve elbow injuries.

24. Bartolo Colon | New York Yankees

Among the major league athletes, Bartolo Colon's stem cell treatment has had some of the most coverage. He was sidelined due to a torn rotator cuff and elbow injury in 2005. He was then one of the first athletes to receive a stem cell transplant on his arm from his fat and bone marrow.

25. Andrew Heaney | L.A. Angels

Andrew Heaney went public about having stem cell treatments in 2016. He had a torn ulnar collateral ligament and received stem cell therapy to aid his recovery.

26. Garrett Richards | L.A. Angels

Garrett Richards had a torn elbow ligament and wanted to start surgery right away. Instead, the team's physical therapist Bernard Li advised Richards to try stem cell treatments. In May 2017, stem cells were extracted from his bone marrow and injected into his elbow.

Leg and Foot Stem Cell Treatments

The four athletes below pursed stem cell therapies to resolve leg and foot injuries.

27. Christiano Ronaldo | Real Madrid

The Real Madrid forward sustained a hamstring injury and tried stem cell treatment to hasten his recovery for their next game in Manchester. The procedure involved harvesting stem cells from his own bone marrow and injecting it into his hamstrings.

28. Ahmad Bradshaw | New York Giants

The Giants running back Ahmad Bradshaw underwent a foot surgery that involved having screws inserted into his foot for two fractures, which he regretted within the year. It wasn't until 2011, when a new fracture occurred, that he decided to seek a different form of treatment. Instead of following through with the surgery, he tried stem cell injections to promote bone regrowth in his foot. In 2012, he had the screws taken out and played for the rest of the season.

29. Prince Amukamara | New York Giants

Prince Amukamara of the New York Giants sustained a broken bone in his left foot from training camp. For bone regeneration, he had stem cells harvested from his bone marrow and injected into his foot.

30. David Payne | Track & Field

The Olympic athlete David Payne suffered a shin injury while he was training for the Olympic trials in 2011. In an attempt to reach his optimum for the trials, he had stem cell therapy with PRP as a regenerative procedure.

Other Types of Stem Treatments for Athletes

The two athletes below pursued other types of stem cell treatments for athletic injuries.

31. Ray Lewis | Baltimore Ravens

Ray Lewis is another high-profile athlete who received a stem cell treatment for a sports-related injury. Lewis traveled all the way to Europe for stem cell therapy on his triceps.

32. Peyton Manning | Indianapolis Colts

The football star Peyton Manning suffered a neck-related injury while playing ball. He traveled to Germany to undergo stem cell treatment, where stem cells from his fat cells were harvested and injected into his neck.

Stem Cell Treatments Beyond Injuries

The six individuals below pursed stem cell therapies for conditions beyond sports-related injuries.

33. Gordie Howe | Detroit Red Wings

The hockey player Gordie Howe experienced a number of small strokes in 2014. At the age of 86, his right side had become paralyzed. Dr. McGuigan from Stemedica, a stem-cell manufacturer, offered Howe and his family an experimental stem cell treatment. The procedure involved millions of neural stem cells injected into his spinal column. He started exhibiting results within days.

34. Jose Contreras | Philadelphia Phillies

Jose Contreras was suffering from chronic pain in his joints and was among one of the first high-profile athletes to try PRP therapy as an alternative to surgery and other invasive procedures.

35. Daisuke Matsuzaka | Boston Red Sox

Daisuke Matsuzaka was the highly fought-for pitcher in 2006. He is also one of the major league athletes who had PRP therapy for painful joints.

36. A.J. Foyt | Nascar Driver

The 82-year-old Nascar driver joined his wife in seeking stem cell treatments to better their health and regain some youth. Foyt had adult stem cells injected into his blood, ankle, and shoulder.

37. Jack Nicklaus | Golf Legend

Jack Nicklaus is a golf legend with 120 professional tournament victories. He went through various medical procedures to help with his chronic joint pain and inflammation. In 2016, he tried stem cell therapy at the Isar Klinikum in Germany. The procedure used liposuctioned abdominal stem cells stained with Matrase to break down the fat tissue.

38. Rafael Nadal | Tennis Player

The tennis player Rafael Nadal had stem cell treatment for back ailments. Stem cells were injected into a joint in his spine to help repair the cartilage. He had also received a similar procedure for his knee the year before.

Published Studies for the Efficacy of Allograft Tissue Products

Derived from Birth Tissue

1. Batsali, A. Comparative Analysis of Bone Marrow and Wharton's Jelly Mesenchymal Stem/ Stromal Cells. Blood.
2013:122:1212.

2. Batsali, AK et.al. Mesenchymal stem cells derived from Wharton's Jelly of the umbilical cord: biological properties and emerging clinical applications. Current Stem Cell Research and Therapeutics. 2-13 Mar: 8(2): 144-55.

3. DiMarino, A. et.al. Mesenchymal Stem Cells in Tissue Repair. Frontiers in Immunology. 2013;4:201.

4. Doi, H. et.al. Potency of umbilical cord blood- and Wharton's jelly-derived mesenchymal stem cells for scarless wound healing Scientific Reports 6 :18844(2016).

5. F Gao et.al. Mesenchymal stem cells and immunomodulation: current status and future prospects Cell Death and

Disease (2016) 7, e2062; doi:10.1038/cddis.2015.327.

6. Hye, J. et.al. Comparative Analysis of Human Mesenchymal Stem Cells from Bone Marrow, Adipose Tissue, and

Umbilical Cord Blood as Sources of Cell Therapy. International Journal of Molecular Science 2013 Sep: 14(9):

17986-18001.

7. Hsieh J-Y, Wang H-W, Chang S-J, Liao K-H, Lee I-H, Lin W-S, et al. (2013) Mesenchymal Stem Cells from Human

Umbilical Cord Express Preferentially Secreted Factors Related to Neuroprotection,

Neurogenesis, and Angiogenesis. PLoS ONE 8(8): e72604. doi:10.1371/journal.pone.007260

8. Kalaszczynska, I and Ferdyn, K. Wharton's Jelly Derived Mesenchymal Stem Cells: Future of Regenerative Medicine? BioMed Research International. Vol 2015 article ID 430847.

9. Liu, Y. et.al. Therapeutic Potential of Human Umbilical Cord Mesenchymal Stem Cells in the Treatment of Rheumatoid Arthritis. Arthritis Research and Therapeutics. 2010; 12(6): R 210.

10. Murphy, M. et.al. Mesenchymal stem cells: environmentally responsive therapeutics for regenerative medicine.

Experimental and Molecular Medicine. 2013 Nov; 48(1) e54.

11. Sobolewski, K. et.al. Wharton's jelly as a reservoir of peptide growth factors. Placenta. 2005 Nov;26(10):747-52.

12. Watson, N. et.al. Discarded Wharton's Jelly of the Human Umbilical Cord: A Viable Source for Mesenchymal Stem Cells. Cytotherapy. 2015 January; 17(1): 18-24.

13. Ye, B. et.al. Rapid biomimetic mineralization of collagen fibrils and combining with human umbilical cord mesenchymal stem cells for bone defects healing. Material Science and Engineering C Material Biology Appl. 2016 Nov 1, 68: 43-51.

14. Bellamy, et al. Viscosupplementation for the treatment of osteoarthritis of the knee. Cochrane Database Syst Rev. 2006 Apr 19;(2):CD005321

15. Didier Demesmin, MD Amniotic Fluid as a Homologue to Synovial Fluid: Interim Analysis of Prospective, Multi-Center Outcome Observational Cohort Registry of Amniotic Fluid Treatment for Osteoarthritis of the Knee Presented at the 2015 AAPM Annual Meeting

16. Brohlin, et al., Characterisation of human mesenchymal stem cells following differentiation into Schwann cell-like cells. Neuroscience Research. 2009, 64(1):41-49.

17. Chaudhury, S. Mesenchymal stem cell applications to tendon healing. Muscles Ligaments

Tendons J. 2012 Jul-Sep; 2(3): 222–229.

18. Udalamaththa, V. et.al. Potential Role of Herbal Remedies in Stem Cell Therapy: Proliferation and Differentiation of Human Mesenchymal Stromal Cells Stem Cell Research and Therapy. (2016) 7:110.

19. Aleynik, et. al. Stem cell delivery of therapies for brain disorders. Clinical and Translational Medicine 2014, 3:24

20. Li, et al., Comparative analysis of human mesenchymal stem cells from bone marrow and adipose tissue under

xeno-free conditions for cell therapy. Stem Cell Res Ther. 2015; 6(1): 55.

21. Anzalone R, et al. Wharton's jelly mesenchymal stem cells as candidates for beta cells regeneration: extending the differentiation and immunomodulatory benefits of adult mesenchymal stem cells for the treatment of type 1 diabetes. Stem Cell Rev. 2011; 7(2):342-63.

22. Tesche LJ, Gerber DA. Tissue-derived stem and progenitor cells. Stem cells international. 2010; 2010:824876.

23. Kalaszczynska, et al., Wharton's Jelly-Derived Mesenchymal Stem Cells: Future of Regenerative Medicine? Recent Findings and Clinical Significance. Biomed Res Int. 2015; 2015: 430847

SOME SUPPORTING RESEARCH for unfocused ESWT:

https://www.softwavetherapy.com/uploads/1/2/1/5/121555836/47._
effect_of_shock_waves_on_macrophages_a_possible_role_in_tissue_
regeneration_and_remodeling.pdf

"Extracorporeal Shock Wave Therapy (ESWT) is broadly used as a non-surgical therapy in various diseases for its pro-angiogenic and anti-inflammatory effects. "

"We can summarize the final effect of ESWT as a general improvement of tissue homeostasis and metabolism, accompanied by improving of the tissue self-healing abilities. Evidence from basic science and clinical studies indicates that this effect involves the ability of shock waves (SW) to support proliferation and differentiation of stem cells, which significantly contribute to tissue healing, but besides stem cells, many other cell targets, including endothelial cells, bone cells, and small unmyelinated nerve fibers, have been involved in ESWT therapeutic potential"

"In most recent years a key role in tissue repair and healing has also been attributed to the innate immunity system, and macrophages in particular play an important role in this setting, both for their key role to control shift from acute inflammation to either its chronicization or resolution phases and for their ability to recruit and stimulate stem cells"

"SW are biphasic high-energy acoustic waves characterized by an initial positive very rapid phase of high amplitude, followed at a distance of microseconds by a sudden phase of mild depression responsible of the biological activity on living tissues. In agreement with the definition proposed by Huang C and collaborators as a therapeutic intervention that reduces and reverse injury to damaged tissues or promotes the homeostasis of healthy tissues by mechanical means at the molecular, cellular, or tissue level SW are today considered a form of mechanotherapy. As for most forms of mechanotherapy in clinical use, ESWT mainly focus on improving tissue regeneration and, consistent with this, clinical results indicate that besides reduction and/or inhibition of apoptosis, the clinical efficacy of ESWT is tightly related to its ability to improve neovascularization and matrix remodeling in tissues."

"The body of scientific data demonstrating that ESWT can induce tissue healing and regeneration through mechano-transduction has brought to the present view of SW as immunomodulators during the wound healing process, which is also well in line with recent evidence indicating that SW influence the TLR3 pathway."

FOR SHOULDERS:

https://www.softwavetherapy.com/uploads/1/2/1/5/121555836/7._eswt_-_calcific_shoulder_2008_mts_orthowave_trt_softwave_.pdf

"In conclusion, the treatment of calcific tendinitis of the shoulder with shock waves has produced a high rate of success in pain relief and functional restoration with negligible associated complications. ESWT is a new therapeutic modality that appears to be both safe and effective for these patients."

https://documentcloud.adobe.com/link/track?uri=urn%3Aaaid%3Ascds%3AUS%3Aefcfda20-1377-40e8-8c69-5b2ad763e402

https://documentcloud.adobe.com/link/track?uri=urn%3Aaaid%3Ascds%3AUS%3A252d16d0-cc3c-4b34-97c1-6f1f86494e24

FOR SPORTS AND AGING POPULATION:

https://www.softwavetherapy.com/uploads/1/2/1/5/121555836/53._ismst_2016_-_key_note_lecture_media_publication_slide.pdf

"Acoustic wave stimulus is seen to:

- Promote tissue regeneration (aberrance rectification)

- Increase tissue resilience – growth facilitation and fatigue resistance

- Improve muscle tone and postural stability

- Similar outcomes are seen in both young athletes and older subjects

- In the athletic population, these outcomes potentially increase career longevity to sports institutions; these outcomes could provide investment security against overuse injuries.

- In the aging population, these outcomes suggest that they could hold a pertinent key to sarcopenia, falls prevention, improved quality of life"

The influence of medical shockwaves on muscle activation patterns and performance in healthy athletes: a preliminary report

https://www.softwavetherapy.com/uploads/1/2/1/5/121555836/10._benefits_of_treating_healthy_athletes_ppp.pdf

Discussion & Conclusion:

From what has been elucidated about the influence of ESWT on tissue suggests:

- Acoustic mechano-transduction influences the cellular-matrix via a myriad of receptors sensory substances

- Promoting favorable cellular communication, interaction and integrity.

- Our investigation suggests that this favorable cascade may not be restricted in pathology but in healthy subjects as well.

- The sustained muscular response and performance improvements (>20 weeks) yielded from this investigation asks the question:

- Can we prevent overuse syndromes by increasing muscle resilience?

- Can we assist athletes in achieving their goals more safely and effectively?

FOR ED (Erectile Dysfunction):

https://www.softwavetherapy.com/uploads/1/2/1/5/121555836/25._case_series_of_weekly_liswt_for_ed.pdf

Conclusion: Once weekly low-intensity shock wave lithotripsy improved erections sufficient for intercourse in 62.5% of our patients without side effects

https://www.softwavetherapy.com/uploads/1/2/1/5/121555836/26._effectiveness_of_swt_in_patients_with_ed.jpg

DEVICES THAT MARKET UNDER SHOCK WAVE THAT ARE NOT

BALLISTIC SHOCKWAVE...Does not produce a shockwave

https://documentcloud.adobe.com/link/track?uri=urn%3Aaaid%3Ascds%3AUS%3A0e4043d4-5b1c-4d4e-82f2-f7f9c2e94bde

"Although the ballistic source investigated marketed both the terms "shock wave" and "focused' the device technically does NOT generate a focused shock wave. Electrohydraulic (EH) sources employ focusing by means of a reflector and generate shock waves at the spark source; for all settings, the EH results in a shock wave at the focus. Electromagnetic and piezoelectric sources also use focusing but do NOT generate shock waves at the source.

RADIAL SHOCK WAVE THERAPY: Does not produce a shockwave at current pressure output

https://documentcloud.adobe.com/link/track?uri=urn%3Aaaid%3Ascds%3AUS%3A30e65f3d-d398-4439-ab8d-6bc6bf54e6a6

"It was shown that shock formation did not occur for any machine settings and that a true shock formation could be reached if the maximum initial pressure output of the device is doubled."

The following studies are for informational purposes only and offer insight into mechanisms of action behind the OrthoGold 100's intended purpose:

https://www.softwavetherapy.com/science.html

NEO MATRIX MEDICAL

WWW.NEOMATRIXMEDICAL.COM

1-855-MATRIX5 (628-7495)

www.ingramcontent.com/pod-product-compliance
Lightning Source LLC
Chambersburg PA
CBHW072105040426
42334CB00042B/2489